The Handbook of Problem-Oriented Psychotherapy

The Handbook of Problem-Oriented Psychotherapy

A Guide for Psychologists,
Social Workers, Psychiatrists, and
Other Mental Health Professionals

A. H. Chapman, M.D.
Miriam Chapman-Santana, M.D.

Jason Aronson Inc.
Northvale, New Jersey
London

Director of Editorial Production: Robert D. Hack

This book was set in 11 pt. New Baskerville by Aerotype, Inc., of Amherst, New Hampshire and printed and bound by Book-mart Press of North Bergen, New Jersey.

Library of Congress Cataloging-in-Publication Data

Chapman, A. H. (Arthur Harry), 1924–
    The handbook of problem-oriented psychotherapy : a guide for psychologists, social workers, psychiatrists, and other mental health professionals / A.H. Chapman, Miriam Chapman-Santana.
        p.   cm.
    Includes bibliographical references and index.
    ISBN 1–56821–682–3 (alk. paper)
    1. Problem-solving therapy.   I. Chapman-Santana, Miriam.
    II. Title.
    RC489.P68C47 1996
    616.89′14—dc20

                                                                95–52522

Printed in the United States of America on acid-free paper. For information and catalog write to Jason Aronson Inc., 230 Livingston Street, Northvale, New Jersey 07647. Or visit our website: http://www.aronson.com

For a dedicated and generous colleague
Djalma Vieira e Silva

Contents

Preface   xi

1   The Therapist's Words and Actions in
    Problem-Oriented Psychotherapy   1

    The Directions in Which Problem-Oriented
        Psychotherapy Moves   6
    Basic Procedures: The Use of Questions   12
    The General Way in Which a Subject Is Explored   17

2   Perception and Nonperception   21

    The Concept of Mentation   24
    Perception and Nonperception in Psychotherapy   29
    Helping the Patient to Construct—and Make
        Sense of—the Story of His Life   32
    The Aims of Problem-Oriented Psychotherapy   36

3 Emotional Pain and the Flow of Communication   39

Emotional Pain as an Obstacle to Understanding
   Everyday Experience   45
Ways of Handling Emotional Pain during
   the Therapeutic Hour   48

4 Emotional Well-Being and Well-Being Operations   55

The Role of Well-Being Operations in Daily Life   56
Healthy Well-Being Operations   57
Unhealthy Well-Being Operations   62
Well-Being Operations Encountered in
   Problem-Oriented Psychotherapy   67
Other Aspects of Managing Well-Being Operations   71
What Is a Personality?   77

5 Making and Testing Tentative Formulations   81

Special Aspects of Verifying Formulations   84

6 Energy Flows in Human Relationships   89

An Example of an Energy Flow in Psychotherapy   92
Other Aspects of Energy Flows in Problem-Oriented
   Psychotherapy   99

7 Distortions and Deviations   101

Distortions as Revealers of Historical Processes   103
The Views of Problem-Oriented Psychotherapy
   on Erotic Developments during Therapy   105
Administrative Manipulation of the Therapist
   as a Deviation in Therapy   109
Factors in the Therapist's Behavior that
   May Influence Distortions in Therapy   111
Temporary Problems of the Therapist that
   May Cause Distorted Reactions in Patients   113

Long-Lasting Problems of the Therapist that
    May Cause Untoward Reactions in Patients   114
The Material Surroundings of Psychotherapy   118

8 Special Techniques   121

Nonverbal Communication   121
Management of Deteriorating Communication   125
Dreams   130
The Use of Humor in Psychotherapy   134
The Patient's Future as an Area for Exploration   138

9 Some Further Aspects   141

To What Extent Should an Interview or a Course
    of Treatment Be Deliberately Organized?   141
Examination of the Patient's View of Himself   146
The Role of Advice   150
Investigation of Abrupt Changes and Gaps
    in the Patient's Life Adjustment   152
The Threefold Nature of Each Person-to-Person
    Relationship   153
Some Broader Aspects of Problem-Oriented
    Psychotherapy   157

10 Problem-Oriented Group Psychotherapy   165

The Basic Types of Group Psychotherapy   165
The Functions of St. Thomas More and
    His Two Wives   166
Murray Steiner's Mission   170
Tandem Polygamy   173
Through a Door, Darkly   175

**11 Combining Psychotherapy and Medications:
A Brief Orientation for Nonphysician
Psychotherapists   181**

Antipsychotic and Antianxiety Medications   182
Clinical and Legal Problems in This Field   186
Disulfiram Therapy   189
Sleep-Inducing Medications   190
A Glossary of Medications Commonly Used
in Psychiatric Disorders   194

References   **207**

Index   **211**

Preface

Every person all his or her life continually encounters and solves problems in his emotional and interpersonal adjustments. One of the newborn infant's first problems is hunger, and he solves it by fretful behavior that brings a breast or a bottle to his lips; his later problems will not be so simply resolved. The complex ways in which a child, adolescent, or adult meets the myriad problems he has with his feelings and thoughts and in his relationships with others are intricate but understandable. In this book we deal with the ways in which problem-oriented psychotherapy can help people in this process. Such therapy focuses on one difficulty after another, clearing the way for sound emotional functioning and healthy interpersonal living. The authors of this book have between them almost seven decades of experience in this kind of work and are hopeful that sharing the results of their successes and failures with you will help to make you a better therapist.

Special mention must be made of the invaluable aid of Simone A. Teixeira, R.N., in drawing up the comprehensive glossary, by trade and chemical names, of medications used in the treatment of psychiatric disorders. This glossary occupies the final two-thirds of Chapter 11, "Combining Psycho-therapy and Medications: A Brief Orientation for Nonphysi-cian Psychotherapists." Ms. Teixeira has so organized this glossary that nonphysician psychotherapists can use it as a desktop reference source when interviewing and evaluating patients who may be taking any of the medications employed in the full spectrum of psychiatric disorders. It also can serve as a ready reference when reading psychiatric articles and books. So far as we know, this glossary, which is both all-inclusive and concise, is unique in books available at this time.

One final note: the principle of indicating the masculine and feminine genders when referring to therapists and others has been maintained at many points throughout the book. However, to do so *each* time this point arises tends to be repe-titious and distracting. The reader should understand the double possibility each time this occurs.

—*A. H. Chapman*
—*Miriam Chapman-Santana*

1 The Therapist's Words and Actions in Problem-Oriented Psychotherapy

An emotionally uninvolved psychotherapist is an impossibility. The therapist who feels he can be a mirror to his patient, reflecting back—and interpreting—the patient's feelings and thoughts without personal involvement, has unjustified confidence in his techniques. A therapist cannot completely control and discount his attitudes and feelings toward his patient. Different patients affect a therapist in different ways; his feelings toward a passive, ingratiating patient and an irritable, contentious one are dissimilar, and from time to time he has a patient who at different points in treatment behaves in both ways. In psychotherapy nothing is static; there is a continual to-and-fro flow of ideas and feelings between patient and therapist. The therapist must steer his patient and himself through this choppy sea, never allowing one or both of them to be tossed about on it.

The therapist is, instead, an *involved sharer*. He shares the patient's experiences, past and present; it is this informed, skillful sharing that makes psychotherapy a unique experience for the patient. Most patients at times share their experiences with other people, but in none of these sharings do they meet with informed, skillful attitudes and reactions. The wife, husband, parent, friend, or co-worker reacts emotionally to what a person says, and as a rule this other person does not do this in an adept way that helps to solve the patient's problems.

General statements like these become clearer if they are illustrated by person-to-person dialogues. Such interchanges must be artificially simplified to make their points in a few words, but they clarify what psychotherapy is all about. Below are two dialogues: in the first the patient is talking with a close person in his life, and in the second one the same topic is dealt with in an exchange between the patient and a therapist.

Person: I've got some bad news. . . . I was fired today. I lost my job.

Wife: Oh my God! Jobs are hard to find right now, and the kids are so young that one of us has to stay at home with them all the time. What happened?

Person: Business is off and somebody had to go. The ax fell on me.

Wife: Didn't they offer you any reason for your being the one that had to go?

Person: No.

Wife: Do you think that they somehow found out about your drinking?

Person: Of course not, and it's not all that big a problem. Anyway, I don't let it affect my work.

Wife: Rob, this is the second job you've lost in less than a year and a half. You've got to do something about your drinking. Everything we have is going down the drain. You just can't go on . . .

Person: Cram it, will you? If it weren't for all the crap I have to put up with here all the time . . .

Wife: Shut up! You just don't want to come to grips with what's happened. You want to go on . . .

Experience is being shared in this interchange but no one is acting in a skilled, informed way. No good, and possibly much harm, will occur if this discussion degenerates into a brawl.

Let us see how this same dialogue, in problem-oriented therapy, might have proceeded in an exchange in which the aim was to help the patient adjust to a critical event in his life.

Patient: I've got some bad news. . . . I was fired yesterday. I lost my job.

Therapist: (*Indicating that he senses the patient's dejection*) That was a blow. Can you tell me how you feel about it and the effect it may have on you and your family?

Patient: I feel like hell. Fran is all upset, and when she's upset the kids are a mess.

Therapist: What did they say at work when they fired you?

Patient: They didn't say anything, but business is off and somebody had to go.

Therapist: Do you think that any other factors influenced their choice of you as the one to be laid off?

Patient: No. This could happen to anybody.

Therapist: Let's look at it from a somewhat different point of view. Sometimes that helps. If you had been your supervisor, would you have explained why this was done?

Patient: I don't know. They never explain things like this.

Therapist: (*Feeling his way along and approaching the same point from a different angle*) Has Fran had anything to say on this score?

Patient: She said what she always says when anything goes wrong.

Therapist: What's that?

Patient: That I drink too much.

Therapist: (*Waits for him to go on. Silence is sometimes the best way to ask a question or make a point; it neither pushes nor accuses the patient. An inquiring but noncensuring facial expression and a slight change in body tone may be important here.*)

Patient: Well, maybe there is something in what she says. Monday mornings are not my best times at work.

Therapist: Perhaps it might be useful to talk a bit more about this, even though it may be painful to do so.

The therapist here has been an involved sharer of the patient's experience and has used informed skill to try to make this interchange—and ones that follow it—useful to the patient.

A quite different kind of life experience is dealt with in the next two dialogues. In contrast to the preceding dialogues, these concern the patient's past rather than his present. The first is with a friend and the second is with a therapist.

Person: Since my father's death six months ago I've found myself thinking a lot about him and me. It goes on all the time.

Friend: You should pull out of this and get interested in other things. You just mope around and you've lost a lot of weight. It's no use going on about something in the past.

Person: I wish I'd made an effort to get closer to him during the last years of his life, especially after we knew he probably had only two or three more years to live.

Friend: He had the best possible care. The doctors saw to it that he didn't suffer much. (*Here the person and his friend are talking on two different levels of experience, and no involved sharing is going on. The friend is distancing himself from the subject to avoid the pain of any real involvement.*)

Person: I was sort of mixed up at the end of my teens. I didn't see things the way my mom and dad did, especially Dad. I guess I didn't know what I wanted, and I'm not sure I do now. I more or less threw it in their faces as well. Sometimes I wonder if all this didn't contribute to my dad's heart trouble. But I can't think about that. That'd drive me nuts. I wish I had it all to do over again.

Friend: Look, you've got to get your mind off this. I'm going to turn on the TV. The game between the Chiefs and the Oilers is about to begin. I'll get some beer from the refrigerator.

As noted, there is no sharing of experience, involvement, understanding, and skillful communication here. The friend, with his "snap out of it" advice, leaves the speaker feeling more isolated and guilty. This is common in nonprofessional discussions of emotional problems.

Let us consider how this same dialogue might have gone on between this person and a problem-oriented psychotherapist.

Patient: Since my father's death six months ago I've found myself thinking a lot about him and me. It goes on all the time.

Therapist: How do your thoughts run?

Patient: Around and around, in circles, all day long.

Therapist: Can you put some of these thoughts into words?

Patient: There're all on the same theme—what might have been, what should have been. They're like corny soap operas with mushy endings. I go over them again and again, adding details. It's pointless. I wish I could turn it off, but I can't.

Therapist: See if you can tell me about one of these scenarios. Sometimes it helps to do so.

Patient: That's what you guys sell, isn't it? And it isn't cheap.

Therapist: (*The therapist at this point identifies and resists a tide of irritability in himself, any expression of which, verbally or nonverbally, would make him useless to the patient.*) Yes, that is what we sell. But we believe in it and we feel that sometimes we help our patients. If one of these scenarios is not too difficult to put into words, give it a try.

Patient: Why not? In one of the corniest of them I go to my dad, put my arm around his shoulder and say . . .

The Directions in Which Problem-Oriented Psychotherapy Moves

A therapist should not assume that all patients who come to him have clear ideas about what occurs in psychotherapy. Sophisticated, well-educated patients usually know these things, but a large number of people in the general public do not. The conceptions a patient may have gotten by seeing psychotherapy portrayed on television or by reading popular books and novels that touch on it often are unrealistic. Some of these difficulties are illustrated in the following condensed patient–therapist interchange.

Therapist: Now that we have covered the main difficulties that bring you to see me—these attacks of marked anxiety, or even panic at times—perhaps we should take a look at what you anticipate will happen in the treatment we are beginning. What are your ideas about how we should go about exploring the causes of this problem?

Patient: Well, talk about my early childhood and what happened then.

Therapist: And only that?

Patient: From what I've read and seen on TV, I guess so.

Therapist: And what about the years and things after that— later childhood, adolescence, adulthood, your marriage, your relationships with your children and with the people at work, and so on?

Patient: Well, maybe they have some importance too.

Therapist: In order to make our work clearer I'll sketch out what we may be concerned with. It isn't so much what happened as what their impacts on you were and the extent to which you were aware of those impacts and were comfortable or uncomfortable with them. We'll be interested in the degree to which you really grasped—that is, could put into words to yourself and to others—what happened in your relationships with the important persons in your life—all your life, from early childhood to the present.

Patient: That sounds like a lot of ground to cover.

Therapist: Sometimes it is. A lot depends on how well we work together. This is a joint venture, a shared exploration.

Patient: I had the impression that psychotherapists more or less know what causes problems like mine and know what to look for.

Therapist: Only in a very broad way. If we knew at the outset what we were looking for and what we should find, it would be a lot simpler, a lot easier. In many cases, moreover, the search is as important as what we find; a lot of work may be devoted to overcoming obstacles to understanding and working out your feelings and thoughts in many relationships with people at various stages of your life.

A basic principle of problem-oriented psychotherapy is *until you find out, you don't know.* If the therapist in the first dialogue at the opening of this chapter had accepted at face value the patient's statement that his discharge from work was due to random chance ("Business is off and somebody had to go. The ax fell on me"), he would have missed the crucial thing in this event.

Finding out, and in the process *sharing with,* is one of the therapist's main activities. Much of the material in this book deals with this process. This of course is not a mechanical procedure, a picking up of stones to see what's underneath. It is more like two people stumbling through the dark with a flashlight that sometimes is bright and at other times is dim.

As a rule, finding out does not proceed toward known goals by questions and probing comments. Systematic goal-directed questioning occurs when a mental health professional is getting information from a patient (and at times from others) whose severe condition makes a rapid evaluation and a sound decision about treatment mandatory. In the majority of cases finding out proceeds by repeatedly approaching many aspects of the patient's experiences by various routes, by withdrawing when one approach is too painful or is otherwise blocked, and coming back to it again by a different path. This is illustrated in the preceding dialogue involving the depressed patient.

It is sometimes argued that if a patient is given enough time in a noncritical, understanding situation, he eventually will do most of this work himself with little intervention by the therapist. We feel that most patients simply cannot talk that well; only sophisticated, strongly motivated persons who come to treatment with well-organized concepts of what therapy should consist of, and where it may possibly lead, can fulfill this criterion. Moreover, problems of time, economy, and third-party payers, such as insurance companies and governments, often interfere with this kind of approach today. In addition, the patient's situation may require quicker action; the first of our two sets of patients above must be helped to become employable, and the second must be helped to emerge from the depths of his depression if the risk of suicide is to be reduced.

Similarly, a therapist should never assume that a patient has understood some important thing that he has said. He must make sure that what he, the therapist, said meant the same thing to the patient that it meant to him. Even individual words, such as hostile, dependent, and passive, may mean quite different things to different people.

For example, in many instances a markedly passive person does not feel that he is passive. He feels that he "likes to get along with everyone," "can't see the point of arguing about things," "never holds grudges," "never met a person he couldn't get along with," and so on. He often feels that these things, regardless of how they are labeled, are valuable personality characteristics and do not constitute a problem that makes him vulnerable to domination and exploitation by others. When a therapist puts together a number of words in a sentence or a small group of sentences the possibilities for the patient's misinterpretation are accordingly greater; the therapist must be certain that what he says really reaches the patient and is assimilated by him.

If a passive person is to make progress, words like passivity and assertiveness must come alive. This is done by examining what occurs in many relationships in his life, often including the one he has with the therapist. Words come alive only when they are related to incidents and relationships in the patient's past and present. For example, his therapy may involve consideration of both small and large things, such as his inability to take defective merchandise back to a store and ask for a replacement, his incapacity to prevent a fellow worker from loading his own work onto him, his reluctance to disagree with his marital partner even when the issue is clear-cut, and many similar things. Only then does the word passive become meaningful and useful to him in thinking about himself. Often he must see that his anxiousness to please the therapist—"to be a good patient," "to bring useful material to each interview," to say things that he feels will indicate to the therapist that he is making progress, regardless of whether he actually is doing so—is a major obstacle in the therapeutic process. In his need to please the therapist he may, in ways of which he as a rule is unaware, avoid talking about important events and relationships and exaggerate the significance of minor ones.

The same is true of many other words mental health professionals use. Words such as hostile, dependent, obsessive, self-defeating, and many others must be explored in many interpersonal contexts in the patient's life. This is fundamental in problem-oriented psychotherapy.

Another principle of problem-oriented psychotherapy is that, as mentioned briefly above, a therapist should not assume on the basis of a patient's symptoms or general clinical picture that a particular kind of emotional trauma in prior years caused this difficulty, or that such symptoms were produced in a narrowly defined, specific span of time during his formative years. For example, a therapist should not posit that an obsessive-compulsive patient underwent, during a one- or two-year period in early childhood, a specific type of conflict with a parent or that he lacked some important kind of emotional experience at that time, the absence of which has marked him ever since despite extensive healthier interpersonal circumstances during most of his years. Life is much more complex, varied, and flexible than such formulations suggest.

The therapist who uses such psychological formulas in attempting to understand his patients will tend to see in them and their past experiences the things he expects to find. In addition he will tend to elicit from the patient material that substantiates his point of view. No problem-solving psychotherapy occurs in these circumstances. In such psychotherapy the patient often brings to the interview material that seems to dovetail with the therapist's theories even when the therapist has not spelled them out to him.

Let us examine how this may occur. Assume that a therapist feels that each painfully shy, withdrawn (schizoid personality) person had during his formative years a tense, cold, rejecting, depreciating mother, and emerged into adolescence and adulthood with an ingrained but inarticulate conviction that all close relationships are traps from which a person rarely escapes, and that minimally comfortable living can be achieved only by emotional withdrawal from people.

As the patient proceeds in therapy he gradually begins to produce life experience data that conforms to the therapist's ideas. When he talks about experiences in which his mother was irritable, rejecting, or depreciating, the therapist is alert and may ask questions or may make brief comments; in other cases the therapist may make nonverbal noises (clears his throat, ceases to cough from time to time, and so on), or may pick up his ballpoint pen and make a note on his clipboard paper. The small noises made by rustling clothing, physical movements and ballpoint pen notations on crinkling paper in an otherwise silent room can be heard by a patient when the therapist is seated outside his field of vision. Such things are of course more easily perceived when the therapist is in front of him, as is more often the case. By these and other verbal (voice tones and pitches are important in this process) and nonverbal cues, the therapist indicates to the patient that this is relevant material. When, in contrast, the patient recounts some incident in which he and his mother had a relaxed good time together the therapist is motionless and silent, and thus the patient in time feels that talking about this second category of experience does not contribute to effective treatment whereas talking about the former kinds of things does. The patient is unaware that he is selecting the data he brings to the interview, and this may begin to happen as early as the third or fourth interview in some cases. Barren, misleading therapy, as opposed to useful problem-solving therapy, is occurring.

In such a case the therapist often gets an unrealistic picture of what happened in the patient's life. If a close friend of the patient's family, or a neighbor who was often in his childhood home, were to enter the therapist's office he or she might say, "Why, that's not the way it was at all. Nancy was a good mother. It was only during the year or so when Larry was ten and she was going through a bad divorce and a rough economic situation for a few months after that that she was tense and couldn't be affectionate to Larry." If the therapist were then to ask this deus ex machina what he or she thought were things that might have damaged Larry he or she might say, "Nancy was unfortunate in her two marriages. Larry's father didn't like kids and showed it, and her second husband brought along a couple of spoiled, demanding boys who monopolized everyone's attention, played Larry off against his parents and pushed him into a corner. When Larry was fifteen Nancy sent him to live with her parents, but by that time he had suffered a great deal and was much like he still is today."

To recapitulate, in problem-oriented psychotherapy, as we shall further discuss in this book, the patient and the therapist engage in an exploration whose course and nature neither of them can foresee.

Basic Procedures: The Use of Questions

Questions as a rule are more useful than declarative statements both to get information and to convey it. If, for example, a therapist says, "She was attempting to break off her relationship with you," the patient can only accept this statement or reject it, saying, "Yes, she was," or "No, I don't think she was doing that." This statement by the therapist puts an obstacle in the way of further exploration of the matter. If, in contrast, the therapist had said, "What do you think she was trying to do when she did those things?" the way is left open for more examination of the event and ones like it.

The more general a question is the better it is. "What were your feelings at the time?" is better than "Did you feel angry at the time?" The first question invites the patient to investigate his feelings, whereas the second one directs his attention to hostile or irritable feelings. Depending on his voice tones and the words he stresses, the therapist by the second question may be more or less telling the patient what his feelings were, or should have been. The patient may not have felt angry; he may have felt abandoned or desolate. A corollary of this principle is that the things a patient finds out for himself in the context of a joint patient–therapist effort are more valuable than those to which a therapist directs his attention by declarative statements or by questions that suggest specific kinds of answers.

One of the most useful questions in a therapist's repertory is "What do you mean by that?" It must of course be asked in a tone clearly implying that the therapist only wishes to understand and is not doubting the truthfulness, accuracy, or frankness of the patient. The same question may be worded "What do you feel that means?" This question is so broad that it more or less is a request to talk further in as open a way as possible. Words that are used in day-to-day speech are better than less frequently employed ones; hence the word *means* in this question is better than kindred words such as signify, imply, or indicate. The last three words sound professorial; they smack of the lecture hall.

Some therapists feel that this kind of close attention to words is irrelevant. It is not. Words and their nonverbal accompaniments are all we have to work with in psychotherapy. One of the central problems in trying to evaluate the methods of twentieth-century pioneers in psychotherapy and to get clear ideas about what actually went on in their therapy (on which they based their formulations and theories) is that we have very little information about what their patients actually said and on the responses or comments the therapists made. For example, these early investigators merely described the Oedipus or other complexes or archetypes that they found in their patients and usually did not specify the things the patients said that led to such formulations. We lack the kinds of data that would allow us to judge for ourselves as objective investigators; in other words, there is little scientific evidence to be reviewed. It is difficult to decide which theories are sound and which are not. As a result, we are left with numerous conflicting theories and methods of psychotherapy and have no truly scientific way of evaluating them. It is as if Newton had written much about the theory of gravity but had never mentioned the apple falling from the tree or analogous things.

Nonverbal features often determine the true nature of a question. For instance, the question "What do you mean by that?" can mean quite different things depending on the words stressed, voice tones, and facial expressions. By "What do you *mean* by that?" the therapist seeks to find out what the patient's opinion of an event was, or what he was trying to say to the therapist. By "What do you mean by *that*?" the therapist is attempting to direct the patient's attention to an unusual, intriguing, or seemingly erroneous conclusion or statement by the patient. By "What do *you* mean by that?" the therapist may be suggesting that other people might feel differently about something.

In addition to their functions in getting information, questions are sometimes the best way of giving it. For example, to a person who is facing an inescapable divorce but is paralyzed by fears that a divorce would damage the children, the therapist may get his point of view across by asking, "Do you think that the short-term distress a divorce would cause would be less traumatic than the damage they are undergoing by being reared in this turbulent marriage?" Somewhat later he may ask, "Is it possible that a divorce would actually come as a relief to the children?"

Many questions should be preceded by well-chosen introductory words as in the following examples. "*I can see why it looks that way to you,* but do your close friends also see it in that light?" "*Since most of the people in your department are worried about the new boss,* is your anxiety about him really abnormal?" "*Let's stand back and look at this;* Has this sort of thing happened to you before, and if so, how did you cope with it?" In each of these three examples the introductory words prepare the patient for what comes afterward; they set the matter in a broader context and indicate that a new approach is about to be used. Such things smooth the flow of an interview and prevent it from seeming to proceed in a choppy way.

In still other cases a therapist may employ questions to urge a patient to explore groundless fears or anxieties. "How did you damage her by saying that?" "Why does a series of events like this indicate that you are incapable of adjusting in a job?" "How many other times in your life have you failed to succeed in a relationship of this kind?"

So far we have been considering *direct* questions. They go straight to the heart of the matter or item being discussed. *Indirect* questions, in contrast, approach a subject or event by seeking detailed information about many aspects of it while the basic point of the subject remains unexamined for the time being. For example, a therapist, in using a direct question may ask, "When you become angry do you tongue-lash people or even at times become physically aggressive?" In employing indirect questions to examine the same subject the therapist would proceed as follows: "Can you think of some particular incident in which you became angry?" "Can you describe in more detail how you felt toward Howard when this happened?" "What did you say?" "What did he say in return?" "What happened after that?" "Did anything else occur as this interchange between the two of you went on?" "How did you feel after you slapped him?" "What was his reaction?" And so on. The therapist and the patient may then go on to explore other relationships in the patient's life in which similar things occurred. In this way the therapist and the patient explore piecemeal this facet of the patient's relationships with people. They do it by examining, one after another, specific things that happened in events in the patient's distant past or recent life.

As a rule the longer such an exploration goes on the more valuable it is in the total process of problem-oriented psychotherapy; there is much more material to work with both at the time and in later interviews. The superiority of this indirect approach to the single direct question, with which we began this discussion, is obvious. This particular series of indirect questions has been artificially shortened for illustrative purposes and we have not dealt with the feelings of anger, vengefulness, shame, or guilt on one side and the possible feelings of shock, resentment, fear, or disgust on the other side. A whole interview might be spent in careful analysis of a single such incident.

Indirect questions in many cases allow a painful subject to be investigated step by step in a way that is more tolerable to a patient. They do not alarm him or assault his self-esteem as the central issue is slowly approached. If the patient begins to be unduly upset as the exploration continues, the therapist can leave the subject, noting to himself and possibly to the patient that it should be investigated at another time in another way.

Loaded questions in most cases should be avoided. A loaded question limits the patient's response and to some extent molds it. For example, a therapist who says, "Why at this committee meeting did you bring up a topic which would probably threaten to break up the session?" indicates the kind of response he expects, or at least influences it markedly. A nonloaded question on the same incident would be, "Why did you say that?" There is, however, an occasional sound use for loaded questions; they may be employed to summarize, at least in part, things the patient and the therapist have been talking about. Thus the loaded question given above might be utilized to summarize a series of events they have been discussing for some time; in such a case the words "as you see it" might precede the rest of the question.

The therapist whenever possible uses *safe* questions. A safe question mobilizes a minimum of anxiety or other emotional discomfort. As we shall discuss in Chapter 3, strong emotional distress tends to block or distort the flow of an interview, and if a patient becomes panicky the interview may terminate altogether. Thus if a therapist inquires, "Did he arouse you sexually when he did that?" he may upset a patient who is not ready to deal with such charged material; the patient may not have been aware of the erotic provocation of his or her companion's act and may be so jolted when it is bluntly pointed out that he veers into a digression or rejects the whole issue with a blanket denial. A safe question to examine the same interpersonal event would be, "How did you feel when he did that?" From that point onward the therapist could feel his way along in investigating the series of verbal interchanges, feelings, and physical acts that occurred, and what their impacts on the patient were.

The General Way in Which a Subject Is Explored

Problem-oriented psychotherapy as a rule begins by examining individual events in the patient's life, one after another. Formulations, definitions of broad problems and conclusions, even tentative ones, are left to a later stage of treatment. A wall is built one brick at a time; though the mason may have a general idea about the eventual form and proportions of the wall, he does not attempt to put on the coping until the wall is well advanced. This is illustrated in the two contrasting patient–therapist exchanges which follow.

Incorrect

Patient: My aggressiveness with people is a big problem.
Therapist: What do you do when you are aggressive?

Correct

Patient: My aggressiveness with people is a big problem.

Therapist: Can you tell me about some incident in which you were aggressive, or felt that you were?

Patient: Well, just last week I blew up at my supervisor when she told me that . . .

As we have noted, problems in living rarely are solved by discussing general subjects like "aggressiveness." They are solved by analyzing many specific interpersonal events in patients' lives and the many complex feelings involved in them.

What is the role of statements, as opposed to questions, in problem-oriented psychotherapy? Declarative statements should mainly be made when all the data supporting them has been marshalled and the statements themselves are virtually obvious. Ideally a statement is made by the patient rather than by the therapist. "I guess I've been manipulating people by making them feel guilty, or upsetting them in some other way, most of my life." "My life is not really the mess I thought it was, though I've had my problems and could have handled a lot of things better."

A certain amount of work should be done in every therapeutic session. Treatment should move along in an uncluttered manner, and digressions that contribute little and minor issues that have already been much discussed should be avoided. In addition, therapy should not be littered with meaningless words such as "I see," "Uh huh," and "I understand." Some therapists feel that these words catalyze treatment, and they do have their place when employed sparingly, but their frequent use annoys or puzzles patients, who feel "If I wanted this sort of thing I could have gotten it by talking to a bartender" or "That's what I get from my husband (or wife) when I'm trying to talk to him and he's half listening to me and half watching television."

Problem-focused psychotherapy does not accept the concept that "mobilizing anxiety" facilitates therapy. Anxiety and other strong emotional discomforts tend to block therapy and to cause profitless digressions as the patient withdraws or shies away from the painful material; they rarely push the patient toward a meaningful consideration of his life. However, if no anxiety, self-loathing, guilt, and other kinds of emotional distress occur during therapy the patient probably is not discussing truly important things. Effective treatment is painful enough as a rule; as one of our patients expressed it, "This is like surgery without anesthesia."

A therapist should make his interpretations and comments concisely and clearly; he should never degenerate into lecturing his patient. He usually can say what he wishes in a few short, well-expressed sentences, and often a single sentence suffices. If a therapist carefully considers what he is saying he usually finds that after a few brief sentences he is merely repeating what he has already said in different words. A patient tends to become uncomfortable when a therapist sermonizes and in many instances simply stops listening. He has had many such discourses from parents, work supervisors, teachers, and others, and the long drawn out interpretation sounds as if he is being "bawled out," "set straight," "corrected," or "told what to do" regardless of the words the therapist uses. It is the length of such an interpretation rather than its content which causes this reaction.

Doing psychotherapy is hard work. It requires constant vigilance and mental exertion. It is the hardest work the authors of this book have known, and each of them early in his or her life did a lot of physical work.

2 Perception and Nonperception

The concepts of perception and nonperception are basic in problem-oriented therapy. A person perceives the nature and meaning of his acts in varying degrees, and in each experience many perceived and unperceived things are continually occurring.

Consider, for example, a surgeon who is removing a gall-bladder. His hands move from one act to another as he separates tissue layers, makes incisions and ties small knots, some of which stop bleeding arteries. As his fingers move deftly in tying one of these knots he does not perceive each nimble movement. He is unaware of them as he concentrates on larger tasks. However, when he was an intern or a surgical resident he did perceive each of the necessary steps in tying a surgical knot as he practiced them on a thread looped over the arm of a wooden chair.

He does not perceive many other things as he performs this operation. He is, on the whole, unaware of the acts of his assistant who shifts a retractor or inserts a suction tip. Similarly, he does not perceive things done by the instrument nurse and the circulating nurse who assist him a short distance away. These things enter his field of perception only if something goes wrong. If the instrument nurse hands him the wrong instrument or if he must ask the circulating nurse to tip the overhead lights slightly the ongoing actions of these people briefly enter his field of perception.

Our surgeon can bring these things into his field of perception effortlessly. He would have more difficulty perceiving many other things about this experience, especially if they were emotionally painful to him. Let us assume that during this operation he is irritable with the intern who is assisting him and snaps at the instrument nurse for the slightest delay, and that this is unusual for him. Various things that preceded this operation cause him to act in this way. Four days before this he was called in consultation on this patient for abdominal pain and felt that the patient had a slight gastrointestinal upset, which palliative medication would resolve. Three hours before the operation the patient arrived desperately ill in the hospital's emergency room and it was obvious that he had a gangrenous or ruptured gallbladder, the consequence of four days' delay in treatment. The surgeon is now engaged in a much more difficult and possibly dangerous operation. He does not perceive that the true causes of his tenseness and irritability lie in his error in diagnosis, and he angrily blames his assistants for any minor or major problem that occurs. The true causes of his emotional state lie in the vast areas of nonperception, which he and every other person have at all times and which include large numbers of past and ongoing experiences.

It is more difficult to bring these things into his field of perception because of their painfulness; they arouse feelings of anxiety, inadequacy, and perhaps guilt. If, however, the patient's family doctor were in the operating room watching the operation he might say, "Relax, Fred. You're upset because you missed this diagnosis four days ago and now have a much more difficult job on your hands. But I agreed with you four days ago; we all make mistakes once in a while." If as a result of his colleague's words, the surgeon relaxes and hence becomes a more effective operator and ceases to bark at his assistants, we might say that the family doctor has had a therapeutic effect on the surgeon; he has had it by moving important emotional material from nonperception into perception.

Let us assume that still other things are active here, and that these things could be moved from nonperception to perception only with much skillful psychotherapy. For example, assume that our surgeon was reared throughout his childhood and adolescence by a harsh, unaffectionate, belittling father and an emotionally indifferent mother and that he emerged into adulthood with strong lurking feelings of inadequacy and battered self-esteem; as a result he has a tendency to feel anxious and guilty whenever things go wrong in his life, especially if his own actions have contributed to them. His current situation has mobilized such feelings in him, though he in no way perceives them, and he in consequence is irritable with his assistants and also is to some extent less adept professionally. Indeed, gnawing feelings of inadequacy and a need constantly to demonstrate to himself and others that he is a worthwhile, achieving person may have contributed to making him a surgeon.

Whether or not this surgeon ever has psychotherapy will depend on many variables. If his current behavior is rare for him, and if his underlying emotional problems are causing him few difficulties in his relationships with his wife, his children, his colleagues, his patients, and his friends, he may never be bluntly faced with the need for psychotherapeutic help. It would enrich his life but it would not be a professional and emotional necessity. On the other hand if experiences such as this ongoing one are common, and if his personality difficulties are contaminating his marriage and his relationships with his children, and if he is by his behavior alienating his colleagues and patients and thus facing professional failure, psychotherapy might be the only thing that could save him from a slow social and economic decline, a marital breakup, and a gradual descent into shabby isolation.

Bringing painful unperceived things into a patient's field of perceived, assimilated, comfortable experience is fundamental in problem-oriented psychotherapy. This process has nothing to do with concepts such as the unconscious mind, unconscious archetypes, unconscious residuals of the birth trauma and other such conceptions, as we shall discuss in the next section of this chapter. Perception and nonperception of past and current feelings, thoughts, and interpersonal events are merely qualities of these things. Just as a feeling may be painful or comfortable, or weak or strong, it may be perceived or unperceived. The facility with which feelings and thoughts, and the memories with which they are associated, may pass from nonperception to perception varies much from one individual to another and from one group of life experiences to another. It also is different at various stages of life. These are major factors in producing emotional health or illness and in determining how well a person makes the constant adjustments that successful living requires.

The Concept of Mentation

Problem-oriented psychology, psychiatry, and psychotherapy do not accept the concept of the mind. If the concept of the mind is carefully examined it is soon evident that it does not lend itself to scientific thinking. Scientific thinking requires that each of its statements, or propositions, is so constructed that it can be proved or disproved by repeatable experiments, which any adequately trained observer can make with the necessary equipment at hand. For example, the scientific concept of gravity can be examined and proved by experiments, which can be repeated any number of times by the same observer and by all other observers.

This is not true of any statement that includes the concept of the mind. For example, consider a simple typical statement about the mind: "Experience is recorded in the mind and integrated with past experience." How can a repeatable experiment, however complex, be set up to test this statement? It is impossible. Experiments can be set up to test such things in *persons*, but persons and minds are immensely different. Moreover it is not permissible to make an unjustified linkage between persons and minds by saying that a mind exists in a person to explain why and how he does whatever he does, because there is no conceivable way of proving or disproving this proposition. To examine a thing one must first localize it, and so vague and elusive a concept as the mind defies localization. In addition, a scientific test requires some kind of sensory perception by an observer who sees or hears something directly or sees or hears it recorded on some type of instrument. There is no possible manner in which sensory perception of the mind (and its actions) can be achieved.

It should be noted here that if a mental health professional worker does not require a scientific basis for his thinking and his work, he is free to use the concept of the mind. But if he does so he should clearly state that his system is based on philosophical reasoning, or simple faith, or commonsense reasoning, or some other system of thought. All these forms of thinking, and any systems of psychology and psychiatry erected by employing them, do not require scientific demonstration. Most of today's mental health professionals, however, are loath to accept anything but science as the foundation for their ideas and work.

What then is the concept of the mind, which all of us use frequently? It is a millenia-old conception, deeply rooted in human thinking, and forms a central feature of philosophical reasoning (sometimes as the psyche), religious faith, theological reasoning, commonsense thinking, and other such systems of thought. It crept into psychology and psychiatry during the nineteenth century and the first half of this century without strict consideration as to whether it conformed to the criteria of science or could be modified to do so. This error has had grave consequences for the evolution of psychology, psychiatry, and psychotherapy.

In considering these things, the brain, an anatomical organ, must not be confused with the abstract concept of the mind. The brain is the central part of a bodywide system, which includes sense perceptors (eye, ear, touch receptors, and others), nerve tracts that carry messages to the brain, and an equally intricate system of tracts that carry messages to the body. The brain also controls or influences functions such as balance, muscular tone, body temperature, heart rate, secretions of hormones, and myriad others. To say that the brain, which cannot be considered apart from this vast network, is the same thing as the mind, or that the mind (an abstract concept in the same sense that the square root of negative one is an abstract concept) is lodged somewhere in this complex and as yet poorly understood organ, is scientifically invalid and involves assumptions that are unjustified at the present time and for the foreseeable future.

The concept of the mind is present in, though less emphasized by, the various forms of psychology, psychiatry, and psychotherapy that have evolved out of Pavlov's conditioned reflex experiments on animals at the beginning of this century. These include, in rough order of their chronological development, behaviorism, learning theory, behavior theory and therapy, cognitive therapy (as it was first presented), and others. Each of them puts emphasis on a central coordinating structure which, if carefully considered, is little more than the concept of the mind decked out in anatomical and biochemical trappings. There is the further and graver question as to whether the results of physiological experiments on lower animals, which lack language and any capacity to form ideas in the human sense of the word, can be extrapolated into human feelings, thoughts, actions, and interpersonal life without unsound assumptions and treacherous analogies so extensive that they take these Pavlov-derived systems far beyond the limits of scientific investigation and fact. It is an immense leap from the conditioned salivation of a dog to the misery of a conflict-ridden marriage, a chaotic adolescent rebellion, suicidal depressiveness, or obsessive-compulsive quandries.

If problem-oriented psychology, psychiatry, and psychotherapy reject the concept of the mind, what do they use to understand human feeling, thinking, and interpersonal life? They rely on the interpersonal acts of people and on the observable feelings and expressed ideas that accompany them. By interpersonal acts we mean activities as diverse as those of a newborn infant seeking a nipple and those of an anxious businessman explaining a new computer system to his recalcitrant staff. Life is a constant stream of interpersonal relationships of myriad natures. Even when he is alone, the thoughts and feelings of a person revolve around things that have happened, or are happening, between himself and others. Even if it seems at first glance that he is not in some way dealing with interpersonal issues, such as when he is working out a problem in mathematics in his study or is daydreaming alone, he is in fact doing mathematics because someone set him to do it or interested him in it, or is daydreaming about something that might occur between himself and others. Every act, thought, and feeling has an interpersonal history—a past, a present, and, possibly, a future.

The things that occur between people can be *observed*. Physical acts can be seen, voices can be heard, physical contacts can be felt, and in rare instances even the senses of smell and taste (as in some forms of sexual behavior) are involved. Modern electronic technology now makes it possible to record ongoing interpersonal relationships on video tapes and other devices. Things that can be so examined can be investigated by more than one observer on the same person as well as on large numbers of people; and, using a little ingenuity, repeatable observations can be set up to test out general statements about what happens in all person-to-person situations. For example, simple experiments can determine if a newborn infant can, after a few weeks, recognize his mother and seek her out from the mass of stimuli that impinge on him; they can determine whether their eyes meet in such contacts, and whether the mother reacts with caring warmth or mechanical indifference. Interesting experiments using these variables have been done to examine what occurs in the early weeks in the lives of children who are later normal or severely autistic. It is much easier to set up experiments on older children, adolescents, and adults, or to catch them as they go about their routine activities, because they have acquired speech, physical agility, mobility, and other social capacities that vastly increase their ranges of observable living.

Thus problem-oriented psychology, psychiatry, and psychotherapy fulfill the requirements of scientific thinking. Their propositions and concepts, always cast in terms of what goes on between people in their immensely varied life situations, can be subjected to observation, and such observations can be recorded for later study. The development of good-quality, easily transported, inexpensive video and audio equipment in the last two or three decades has moved the entire field of problem-oriented psychiatry into the realm of practical experimentation.

The presence of the concept of the mind in twentieth century psychology, psychiatry, and psychotherapy has had marked effects on the evolution of these fields; from our point of view these effects have been mainly undesirable. Because systems of psychology and psychiatry founded on the concept of the mind are constructed of statements that can be neither proved nor disproved, the way for proliferation of one psychiatric and psychological system after another, each claiming to be the only valid one, is made possible. Thus modern psychiatry is filled with a bewildering array of competing schools—Freudian, Jungian, Adlerian, Rankian, Horneyan, Kleinian, Lacanian, Gestalt, Rogerian, and others. One observer summarized this situation in his statement that "Once you accept the idea of the mind, often with divisions into unconscious, preconscious and conscious parts, you can arrange the furniture in it any way you want, and no one can prove that your system is any better, or any worse, than anybody else's arrangement."

Perception and Nonperception in Psychotherapy

One of the fundamental tasks of problem-oriented therapy is to help the patient perceive the nature and meaning of what is going on in his or her life, and what has gone on in the past. In this process feelings, thoughts, and interpersonal acts move from the realm of nonperception into the area of perceived, assimilated experience. This is much more than merely "finding out" or "seeing for the first time." The gradual incorporation of new ways of looking at one's life, of assimilating old unperceived things into more meaningful living, and of the evolution of sound personality patterns to replace unhealthy ones, are all involved in the process designated by the word *perceive*. This is illustrated in the following condensed, simplified patient–therapist dialogue.

Patient: Bob told me time and again that the contraceptive pills I was taking were making me irritable and quarrelsome.

Therapist: Did he suggest that you stop taking them?

Patient: Not exactly. He just said that they were upsetting me and fouling up our marriage.

Therapist: Did you see it that way?

Patient: We were arguing a lot more.

Therapist: About what sorts of things?

Patient: He complained about the meals. He said we always had the same old things, meals you heat up in the microwave or put in the oven for a short time.

Therapist: What did you think about these complaints?

Patient: I don't know. He was very insistent about them.

Therapist: How long had you been making meals this way?

Patient: Ever since we got married.

Therapist: Would it be fair to say that the change was in his opinion about the meals rather than in the meals themselves?

Patient: I guess so. Nothing had really changed much.

Therapist: Was he fussy and hard to please about other things?

Patient: He began to be. Up until then he hadn't paid any attention to whether or not the apartment was in a mess, and whether the bathroom looked as if a cyclone had gone through it. There had always been dirty clothes in corners and books and papers piled on the chairs and the sofa. He hadn't ever complained about any of that.

Therapist: Did he make suggestions about how the meals might be changed and about what might be done about the apartment in general?

Patient: He wanted me to stop buying ready-to-heat food. He even bought me a copy of *The Joy of Cooking* and pointed out a lot of recipes in it, and said I ought to organize the apartment better.

Therapist: Anything else?

Patient: He said we ought to have a clothes hamper for dirty clothes and that I might wash some of them myself, the lighter things, rather than, as he said, throw all that money away at the laundromat. And other things.

Therapist: How would such changes have altered your life?

Patient: I didn't see how I would have time to go on working on my degree and writing my thesis if I did all those things, or even some of them.

Therapist: Did you tell him that?

Patient: Yes, but he just said that if he had wanted to live like we were living he wouldn't have gotten married.

Therapist: Did discussions about these things occur often?

Patient: More and more, until we were arguing about them every day.

Therapist: What do you think was going on here? What was he *really* driving at?

Patient: I don't know.

Therapist: How did you *feel* about these problems?

Patient: In time I got scared.

Therapist: Scared?

Patient: Worried. Apprehensive.

Therapist: Worried about what?

Patient: I knew I couldn't complete my degree if I did all the things he wanted, and I still had almost two years more to go.

Therapist: Did it seem, as time went on, that the situation was pushing you to a choice?

Patient: Yes. He finally began to ask me which was more important, our marriage or my degree.

Therapist: How did you *feel* about this?

Patient: More scared. The last thing I wanted was a broken marriage. I'd seen my parents go through one after another of them, and all my life I'd sworn not to have a life like that.

Therapist: And through all of this did Bob persist in saying that the basic issue was your emotional tension and quarrelsomeness caused by contraceptive medication?

Patient: Yes. I got increasingly upset. Depressed. Maybe a little desperate. So I finally stopped taking the pills and before I got the money together to go and have an IUD put in I got pregnant. Bob wouldn't hear of an abortion. A few months later I dropped out of school. Froze my studies and got a long extension on my thesis.

Therapist: When you began to devote yourself to household tasks and dropped out of school and had the baby, did Bob seem more satisfied?

Patient: Yes. Everything settled down.

Therapist: And how did *you* get along in this new way of life?

Patient: I was unhappy. I had saved my marriage, but it didn't seem to end my anxiousness and depressiveness. But I covered up in front of Bob.

Therapist: Anxious about what? Depressed about what?

Patient: I was now totally dependent on Bob. If anything happened to our marriage I could only go back to selling Avon products door to door, or something like that. And now there were two of us, the baby and me. It was my mother's life all over again.

Psychotherapy is possible because a patient communicates more than he or she realizes. The therapist helps the patient to enlarge his perception of his life experiences. Feelings, thoughts, and interpersonal events, with their significance and ramifications, move from the realm of nonperception into perceived, assimilated experiences.

The patient then has what he or she needs to adjust more comfortably and effectively to his life circumstances. He also has acquired a new way of looking at his difficulties that will stand him in good stead for later, different problems.

Helping the Patient to Construct—and Make Sense of—the Story of His Life

One of the tasks of problem-oriented therapy is to help the patient see how the major interpersonal relationships of his life have molded his personality and have made him the kind of person he is. It should be noted here that we believe the elucidation of the human genome by ongoing DNA studies is probably going to change this only to a limited extent. The influence of past and present environment on character structure and emotional problems is, moreover, the only part that both the patient and his therapist can do something about. For the patient in front of you, with his day-to-day anguish and dilemmas, his DNA structure is water under the bridge. Sometime late in the next century this situation may conceivably be different, but the authors and readers of this book will then no longer be around. We must deal with things as they are, not as they may be in the distant future.

Therapy in a sense helps the patient to construct the story of his life and to make sense of it. This is done, in the final analysis, by careful attention to endlessly large numbers of details. These in time lead to consideration of the ways in which the patient adjusts, or fails to adjust, to people who attempt to manipulate him, or to dominate him, or to arouse him erotically, or to panic him into certains kinds of action, or to influence him in other ways. For example, in the dialogue above, which begins with day-to-day details such as meal preparation and household tasks, it becomes clear that the patient adjusted badly to the attempts of her husband to manipulate her into becoming dependent on him, and that this maladjustment was rooted in her desperate need to avoid a pattern of successive marital failures similar to those that had occurred in her mother's life.

How does a therapist distinguish important details from unimportant ones? Important details as a rule are identified by the nonverbal clues that accompany them. Such things as whether a patient's facial muscles become taut when a subject is mentioned, or whether he has a slight change of voice tone, or becomes physically restless, or whether an unusual gesture occurs, alert the therapist to the fact that something notable has been touched on. In other cases the patient may stumble

over words, or try to push a topic aside, or attempt to camou-
flage it with a stream of irrelevant chatter, or laugh inap-
propriately, or lapse into silence. Much time in the training of
psychotherapists, perhaps with the aid of audio and video
tapes, should be spent in developing sensitivity to these signs.
A significant detail usually is connected in some way with what
is going on, or has gone on, in the patient's relationship with
some close person in his life.

There are three general stages in the examination of each
topic or each aspect of a patient's life. The first is the establish-
ment of data. What happened? How did it happen? What
emotions were associated with the event? What further facts
are needed to understand it better? This is illustrated in the
following patient–therapist interchange in which a small detail of an interpersonal incident is explored.

Patient: And then my mother left the room.
Therapist: (*Noting that the patient became a little tense as he said
this*) Where did she go?
Patient: Into the kitchen.
Therapist: Did she come back?
Patient: No.
Therapist: Did she continue the conversation from her new
place in the kitchen?
Patient: No.
*A period of silence occurs as the therapist waits for the patient to go
on; since he does not, the therapist speaks.*
Therapist: Could you now see her from your position in the
breakfast room and could she see you from her place in the
kitchen?
Patient: No. She closed the door as she left.
Therapist: (*Again noting a vague discomfort in the patient as he
said this*) Closed the door?
Patient: Yes.

Silence. (Such resistant or evasive silence is unusual for this patient; the therapist notes this.)

Therapist: Does your mother usually close the door as she goes from one room to another?

Patient: I guess not. I suppose she wanted to make a point. She didn't want to discuss this subject anymore.

Therapist: In making her point was it necessary to do more than simply to leave the room?

Patient: It was the way she did it.

Therapist: The way she closed the door?

Patient: She slammed it. Hard.

An important detail has been brought out, and it quite possibly is the most significant one in this incident. It perhaps tells something about the mother's personality and the ways in which she relates to the patient, and maybe to other people.

The second stage of problem-focused psychotherapy begins after many facts have been established. It consists of the formation of a hypothesis about some aspect of the patient's life; as a rule it deals with some facet of his ways of adjusting in interpersonal situations. For example, in the case of the patient in the preceding dialogue, after establishing a great deal of data about what had gone on and was still going on between him and his mother, the therapist might say, "In doing these things and behaving in this way, perhaps your mother was trying to prevent you from moving out of the house and becoming independent."

In the third stage of therapy the general formulation, or hypothesis, is examined to determine whether it is valid or not. Every formulation is tentative in the beginning. As a rule this process of verification proceeds by exploration of many other relationships and incidents in the patient's life. Do similar things happen in his relationships with friends, casual acquaintances, co-workers, and supervisors? Do they

occur particularly with women or with men, or equally with
both men and women? Is there something in his personality
that leads him to avoid people who tend to manipulate him in
this way, or, in contrast, to drift into relationships repeatedly
in which he is exploited? What emotions—such as anxiousness, guilt, shame, or others—occur in the various stages of
such a relationship? In time a new insight is consolidated and
the patient's interpersonal activity and ways of feeling and
thinking change. He begins to adjust better, through both
changes in himself and the alterations he makes in his interpersonal circumstances.

In a sense the therapist helps the patient write the story
of his life, or some significant segment of it. As he looks back
at his life he sees how unsatisfying—or, frankly, sick—
relationships have hampered him, how he repeatedly has
done self-defeating things, and how former relationships and
events have led to later difficulties. The sound areas of his life
are also noted, but because they are not causing his problems,
much less time is spent on them. When he can assimilate these
things, his life, or at least important parts of it, no longer
seems to have lurched haphazardly from one episode to
another and from one unhealthy situation to the next. His life
makes sense. Causes, effects, and progressions of events become clear; every interpersonal pattern or personality characteristic has its history. This may be a painful process, but the
way is now open for more comfortable, effective living. The
patient is freed from the unhealthy parts of his past, and from
this point onward, he can adjust better to life's continual opportunities and difficulties.

The Aims of Problem-Oriented Psychotherapy

The best criterion of a person's emotional and interpersonal health is the extent to which he or she is aware of the

nature of his feelings, thoughts, and interpersonal patterns in the many situations of his day-to-day life. A person who has such broad insight is as a rule little troubled by problems in living; he rarely is psychiatrically ill.

Everyone wants to live comfortably and effectively. Everyone wants to be as free as he can be of emotional pain—anxiety, guilt, depressiveness, self-loathing, eerie sensations, and others—and he wants relationships that are satisfying. He wants to get along well in each new life situation and he wants affection and harmony in both his close relationships and his broader social, economic, and cultural ones. This is the driving force behind psychotherapy. To the extent that a person achieves these things in treatment, he becomes healthier.

Improvement begins in the treatment situation; from there it spreads outward into the patient's life. Consolidation and extension of a patient's gains occur in his daily experiences during the time he is in treatment and go on long after therapy ends; in many cases these processes continue for the rest of his life. Psychotherapy cannot eliminate problems in a patient's life; for new problems, both large and small, are inevitable as time proceeds. After successful treatment, however, a patient has enhanced abilities to encounter and solve these problems and to achieve better adjustments, in the broadest sense of the term.

3 Emotional Pain and the Flow of Communication

Emotional pain includes all forms of distress in feeling—tenseness, fearfulness, anxiousness, panic, feelings of personal worthlessness and inadequacy, guilt, shame, self-loathing, eerie sensations of changes in oneself or one's environment, and other kindred sensations. It may vary in degree from scarcely noticeable discomfort to disorganizing panic.

Such a neat classification of emotional distress is always a little artificial. The person who is suffering from it has two or more of these discomforts in any episode of emotional upset and often cannot describe well, both at the time and afterward, what he was feeling. Whenever the term emotional pain is used in this book it should therefore be understood that a complex form of anguish is being discussed.

Emotional pain hinders communication in a patient–therapist relationship and in all other person-to-person situations in which it occurs. One of a therapist's tasks is to keep the level of emotional pain down to a point at which it is not a hindrance to communication. The way in which emotional distress obstructs communication is made clear in the following analogy. If during an interview a patient has a sudden bout of severe abdominal pain due to spastic colitis, he is unable to continue talking about his life experiences. If a short time later the pain subsides, he can return to exploring his interpersonal and emotional life, but he remains uneasy and his attention is easily distracted because he fears that at any moment his physical pain might return. Emotional pain acts similarly. It is an even greater deterrent because emotional pain is precipitated by the interview process itself, and the patient usually grasps this fact. As a result, he may veer away from discussing whatever he was talking about when the emotional pain began; he may deviate by discussing irrelevant topics or flooding the interview with banal chatter. In rare instances panic terminates an interview altogether. We remember a 19-year-old patient in the early years of our work who, when a highly charged subject was broached, rose and ran from the room, never to return again.

On the other hand, if no emotional tension occurs during psychotherapy, it is probable that significant things are not being discussed. The therapist must be constantly alert to detect emotional distress and to evaluate whether it is a sign that important things are being discussed or a signal that a topic is too charged to be examined at that time.

Patient: . . . and on Friday morning I got a telephone call from Barbara Holmes. She was all upset. She'd discovered that her husband has been going out with some girl who punches a computer in his office, and when she confronted him with it they had a terrible fight and he ended up asking for a divorce. And they've been married for almost thirty years. Mark Holmes is the last man in the world whom you'd imagine doing a thing like this.

Therapist: Did Barbara's telephone call upset you too?

Patient: Mark Holmes was only an auto parts salesman working for McKinley and Stephens, taking orders from garages
and dealers in small towns twenty-five years ago. Then he
started his own business and began to import auto parts
from places like Korea and Taiwan. He's now one of the
biggest dealers in this part of the country. He undersells
everybody. That's one of the big things that's wrong with
this country, flooding the market with all kinds of things
made in nations where labor is cheap. I think the President
and the Congress are all wrong about . . . (Continues for
two more minutes in this vein).

Therapist: (*Noting that the patient, with a tense urgency of speech,
has turned away from the subject in hand and has talked about
something remote from it and from her life*) Is there something
about the breakup of the marriage of this middle-aged
couple that particularly disturbs you?

Patient: This sort of thing could never happen in our family.
My sister's marriage is as sound as a rock and my brother is
an ideal family man. In February he and Martha are going
to take a Mediterranean cruise. They go aboard in Genoa,
sail down the coast, go inland to see Florence and Rome,
and then . . . (Once more the patient veers abruptly away
from the topic under consideration and spends a few minutes on an irrelevant subject. This is unusual for her in
therapy.)

The therapist of course has noted the patient's two anxious
flights from the subject of marital infidelity and breakup:
first into the details of Mark Holmes's business career and
then into the itinerary of a cruise her sister and brother-in-
law are going to take. If the patient had continued longer in
either of these digressions the therapist would have been
forced in some adept manner to prevent therapy from being
paralyzed for the rest of the session, or for a large part of it.
He must now decide whether to explore the patient's own

marriage for evidence of similar stresses or, feeling that this area is too upsetting for current examination, lead their dialogue into some less disturbing area for the time being. He might approach this anxiety-ridden matter later by investigating the ongoing adjustments of the patient's two late-adolescent children to see if these adjustments have recently deteriorated, and if that deterioration is associated with things their father is doing that gravely affect their parents' marriage. This is only one of several ways by which this painful area could be approached in a manner less upsetting to the patient. A rising titer of anxiety in the patient has here been a hindrance, hopefully temporary, to the therapeutic process.

In the following patient–therapist dialogue the therapist is successful in (a) reducing the patient's level of emotional distress and (b) then using this as an opportunity to investigate an important facet of the patient's life.

Patient: I don't feel anything in sex anymore. It doesn't turn me on. I'm avoiding it. Whenever Bill wants sex, and he wants it every day, I find other things to do. I go into the kitchen and make something, or stuff some clothes into the washer, or tidy up the apartment. It's bothering Bill a lot.

Therapist: When did this begin?

Patient: Right after we got married four months ago. And I couldn't get enough of it with Bill before we got married. We always went to a motel first thing when he came to town and I enjoyed it, and it was like that every day. I thought that after we got married and were always together I'd want it a lot. I can't understand what's happened to me.

Therapist: Are you worried that from now on sex is going to be always like this?

Patient: Yes, and Bill's beginning to think the same thing. He wants to know if I still love him, and I do. That's not changed.

Therapist: (*Moving to reduce the level of the patient's emotional distress as the first step in exploring the general subject of married life and the role of sex in it*) The chances that your sexual adjustment will gradually return to its former state are good. When a person has had a good sexual adjustment and a problem like this—indifference or rejection in a woman or impotence in a man—occurs, the previous level of sexual adjustment almost invariably returns gradually. This occurs with or even without treatment. When the job is to create a level of sexual activity that a person has never had, in either a woman or a man, the process is much more difficult and the percentages go down.

Patient: Can I count on that?

Therapist: Yes, the statistics, to use a cold word, are strongly on your side. (*Now that the patient's anxiousness is reduced and she can talk more freely on this broad subject, he begins to explore this facet of her life.*) What does sex, as an important experience, mean to you?

Patient: It's what cements a man and a woman together. Without it love doesn't last.

Therapist: Are you worried that if this goes on and on your marriage will break up?

Patient: Yes. (She starts to cry.)

Therapist: (*Again diminishing her emotional pain to permit a meaningful exploration of this area to proceed*) To repeat, this problem is usually sure to recede and your good sexual adjustment with Bill will return. I have a lot of experience to back this up and I can show it to you written in books as well.

Patient: I believe you.

Therapist: Let's look at this more broadly. Everyone is an expert on one marriage, the one he or she was reared in, the marriage of his parents. What was the general emotional atmosphere in your parents' marriage, and the implied sexual relationship in it?

Patient: It wasn't good. In fact it was awful. When I was eleven one of my girl friends told me that my father showed her his genitals when they were alone together in the kitchen. I couldn't believe it. I told my mother what she said and Mom said that Dad had this problem and that it caused a lot of trouble from time to time. The police had had complaints and they had hauled him into court three times; once they forced him to go to a psychiatrist but he didn't stick to it and nothing came of it.

Therapist: Did this painful problem intrude on your own life more times after this episode with your girl friend?

Patient: Yes, four more times. The last was when I was sixteen. He did it in the car twice when driving one of my friends home and a couple of times even in the living room when no one was there but him and the girl. I wondered how many other times it happened and the girls didn't tell me, and perhaps told no one. There were girls who stopped coming to our house for no apparent reason. It was like living on a volcano; you never knew when it was going to erupt and ruin everything. I talked to Mom about it. She said he promised time and again to stop it, and sometimes he did for a while, but then it started happening again. It all came to a head when the man next door wanted to kill him, or at least to beat him up badly, because he did it a couple of times in front of this man's wife. There was a terrible uproar. When I was seventeen my parents were divorced.

Therapist: Sex, in your life after the age of eleven, was hence a painful, destructive thing. It contaminated marriages and homes and broke them up. It was a nightmare rather than a loving, unifying force.

Patient: Yes, I guess so.

Therapist: And this was *married* sex. It was sex that occurred after people got married and set up a home, as opposed to sex before marriage.

Patient: Yes.

Therapist: I think this is an important aspect of your life and it probably plays a large role in your current sexual problem. It may also contribute to the persistent, repetitive, upsetting thoughts and the endless checking and rechecking of things at home and at work that brought you to see me. I think we shall have to spend a lot of time talking about all aspects of this, even though it may hurt a good deal.

Patient: It's good to get it out into the open with someone. You're the first person I've ever told this to, except Mom. But she wouldn't really discuss it. She just said it was a sickness in him. It was a big factor in causing their divorce. Even Bill knows nothing about this. I've never told him.

To recapitulate, the therapist here has first reduced the level of the patient's emotional distress. If he had not done so it might well have been an obstacle to exploration of an important sector of her life, and might have caused treatment to become a sterile process. He secondly has taken advantage of the reduced titer of emotional pain to approach this area.

Emotional Pain as an Obstacle to Understanding Everyday Experience

Emotional pain, especially when it is severe, hinders the perception and understanding of experience in day-to-day living. A person in a panic state may be more or less unaware that an automobile accident has occurred a short distance away from where he is standing, and a profoundly depressed person may not perceive that someone in the same room with him has dropped a cup of coffee or is behaving in a crude manner. In terms of the assimilated experience of the panic-ridden or depressed person, it is as if these things had not occurred; later he may remember them imperfectly or not at all.

In a similar way many things do not enter the awareness of an individual in a lesser state of emotional pain. He may not perceive that someone is angry at him, or is cold and rejecting to him, or is attempting to flirt with him. It is as if the angry, cold, or flirtatious person were doing nothing of note in regard to him. These persons are perceived only as a chair or a table in the room is perceived; they make little or no emotional impact on him.

A major task of psychotherapy is to help the patient to become aware of what is going on emotionally in his life and to recapture much of what has occurred in the past. Until these things are included in his fund of comfortable, assimilated experience they cannot be used to solve his problems and to live in more effective ways.

The therapist thus is often faced with the problem of missing data. Effects are present without apparent causes, and causes without effects are encountered. It is as if the patient and the therapist were attempting to put together a jigsaw puzzle with half the pieces missing. Often the therapist must reflect to himself, and perhaps to the patient, "But this account is incomplete. A lot of things are missing." Frequently the therapist can make astute guesses about the nature of the missing information, but so important a thing as personality health cannot be constructed on a foundation of assumptions and guesses, no matter how sagacious. The missing feelings, thoughts, facts, and interpersonal nuances must be found.

This is done by approaching the matter or event under consideration in as many ways as possible. As an example, let us consider time sequences. The therapist at times reflects (usually to himself, but sometimes to the patient), "But that must have happened long after this incident. The patient is bringing into an event in his late adolescence things that could only have happened during his childhood." Or, "She could not have felt this way toward him at that point; the breakup of her family had not yet occurred." In such circumstances the therapist may refer to other participants in the event as observers. "What does your wife remember about this trip to New Orleans? Has she ever talked about what happened there and how it affected you?" or "Has your brother ever talked about that summer when your mother had the automobile accident?"

A sequence of such questions, much simplified and shortened here for purposes of illustration, might proceed along the following lines: "Does your sister remember your mother's death? She must have been about 18, and you were 14, when she died. Has she ever talked about the trip to the psychiatric hospital in Portland which your father and the two of you made a few weeks before she died? From the few things you do remember about that trip, such as the water cooler and the plastic cups in the hall outside her room and the agitated old man shouting incomprehensible things while his wife and son tried to calm him, you apparently went to the floor where your mother was. Does your sister recall whether you went into her room or stayed outside while she and your father saw her? It is not clear whether your one poignant memory of her, lying in bed silhouetted against a large window with bare tree branches outside, is actually from this hospital visit or from some earlier time in your life. Does your sister remember her in this way? We would like to understand why this memory haunts you so much that it blocks out almost all other memories of your mother." This exploration in actual therapy would of course stretch over an entire interview, or perhaps several interviews.

Beyond the bare facts of this experience, and of all human experiences, lie the feelings and painful thoughts associated with them. In addition to their own importance, feelings are significant as the factors that made this event so painful a tableau that the patient has little recollection of what actually occurred in it. In investigating these things many forms of experience may be used. Dreams and dream fragments, especially if they are upsetting and recurrent, sometimes elucidate such interpersonal events. At times the patient's symptoms—his obsessive thoughts or compulsive acts and rituals, or his phobic or depressive ruminations, or other symptoms—may point to what occurred and can accordingly be analyzed. Slips of the tongue, special attitudes toward certain groups of people, and habitual gestures or facial expressions when charged topics are under consideration, may be helpful. Also, tendencies in thinking, such as rapid jumps to unjustified conclusions, or the inability to see obvious relationships, or ingrained pessimism or optimism about one or many things in life, may give useful information. The kinds of reading, television and video programs, and music the patient finds pleasant or repulsive sometimes aid in this process. Proclivities to overuse certain words (we recall a patient who tended to classify many things as "potent" or "not potent") and many other things may contribute to the therapeutic work in this regard.

As a result of such therapy the patient acquires a much larger fund of digested, comfortable experience to help him as he adjusts to the current and future opportunities and problems of his life.

Ways of Handling Emotional Pain during the Therapeutic Hour

A therapist cannot effectively reduce emotional pain until he knows what the patient is distressed about. It is insufficient to say, "Depression like this is common," or, "A certain amount of tension, or even severe anxiety, often occurs in people." It is far better to specify, at least in general terms, the cause of the emotional discomfort and to link it to something in the patient's ongoing or past experiences. "Depression like this is common as a person surveys his life, which, as he sees it, is filled with failures." "A certain amount of tension, or even severe anxiety, often occurs in a person as he contemplates his first steps in being more assertive with people who take him for granted and may be dominating and exploiting him."

If the therapist is unsure what the patient is feeling anxious, or guilty, or inadequate about, he should try to find out before commenting on the emotional pain itself. This may require a brief or prolonged exploration of current or past events and relationships. There are, however, some exceptions to this general principle. In some cases investigation of the things to which emotional pain is linked entails the risk of precipitating panic or marked depression. An adolescent boy or girl who is alarmed, often in inarticulate ways, about homosexual impulses in himself or herself may be panicked by such an exploration. In such cases it is best to go slowly into this area or to put it aside altogether for the time being. "It's not important that we go into this at this time. Another time, when we've solved other difficulties, will do just as well." These instances, however, constitute a minority of situations in which emotional turmoil occurs during the therapeutic hour. In most instances it may be investigated without danger.

In many cases the cause of emotional discomfort that occurs during the therapeutic hour can be ascertained by glancing back at what has been discussed during the preceding minutes or during the entire session up to that point. This happens in the following abbreviated patient–therapist dialogue.

Patient: This is the promotion I've waited for for years, but now that it's come I don't seem to relish it, and that bothers me. I seem to want to put it off, and it can't be put off. I feel sort of tense and down in the dumps, and I should feel the exact opposite.

Therapist: Perhaps if we take a backward glance at what we've talked about in this session we can begin to see why the promotion has lost its attraction for you and actually seems to upset you as you talk about it.

Patient: You mean about Montgomery being edged out and me getting his job.

Therapist: How do you *feel* about this?

Patient: He hasn't adjusted to the new system. He never liked computers when they were first installed about ten years ago and he hates this new generation of computers, word processors, and software that's coming in now. He doesn't really understand them and what they signify. Down deep he longs for typewriters, filing cabinets, in-trays and out-trays and all the paperwork that goes with them.

Therapist: And you?

Patient: I'm with it. I can handle it all and I see that it's a big step forward. The head people in our division know that I understand it all and that Montgomery has dragged his feet. They know I've taken a lot of courses and other training during the last year and a half, and at my own expense. They see that I'm the logical one to fill Montgomery's place.

Therapist: How did the head people know about your special training if the company paid for none of it?

Patient: I talked to people and knew the news would filter upward. When the computer institute held its graduation exercises I put the bosses on the list of people I wanted invitations sent to.

Therapist: How old is Mr. Montgomery?

Patient: Fifty-two. But that's not the point. It's the age of your thinking and not your age in years that counts.

Therapist: Did Mr. Montgomery know you were taking these special courses?

Patient: Probably not, until the end. I saw no point in telling him.

Therapist: What is Mr. Montgomery going to do when he leaves the company next week?

Patient: I don't know. Jobs aren't easy to find when you're his age. He has a brother who has a travel agency in Pentonville and he's talked about going there. Maybe that's what he'll do.

Therapist: A travel agency in Pentonville can't be very big.

Patient: I guess not. He should have kept up with the times.

Therapist: Is there something about taking Mr. Montgomery's situation that bothers you? Is it that, rather than the job promotion itself, that is in some way making you uncomfortable?

Patient: My sister says I'm a sort of hatchet man in this.

Therapist: What do you mean by hatchet man?

Patient: A guy who does somebody else in. But my sister's got it all wrong. I didn't do Montgomery in. He did himself in. He's got other problems. A salesman who sometimes comes into the office and who knows him pretty well says he's begun to hit the bottle lately.

Therapist: Does your sister have anything else to say about this?

Patient: She says that this is more or less what happened to our Dad when he was in his fifties. But God damn it! I'm not responsible for Montgomery's problems. What the hell can I do about them? Somebody had to get his job. So why not me? If a man can't . . .

The therapist and the patient, working together, have identified the thing to which the patient's anxiety and depression, and possible guilt feelings, are linked. The patient has made this connection without a specific interpretation by the therapist. However, his ensuing agitation indicates that they have gone far enough for the present; some therapists might feel that they have gone too far.

The therapist here has found several areas that probably will have to be approached later. To what extent was Mr.

Montgomery a father figure to the patient? What happened to the patient's father in his middle-aged vocational crisis, and how well did he adjust to it? What effects did the father's job crisis in middle age have on the patient, who was either in the last years of high school or in college at the time? Does the patient, in this connection, sometimes glance forward toward his own middle age some twenty-odd years down the road? These are areas that can be addressed one by one and at a later time in treatment. At the end of this dialogue the therapist directed the course of the interview into a less stressful channel.

A final aspect of this patient–therapist dialogue should be pointed out. There is an error of technique in it. The patient always refers to the middle-aged man whom he is replacing as "Montgomery," whereas the therapist repeatedly calls him "Mr. Montgomery," giving him an implied consideration and prestige that the patient does not. This, probably combined with compassionate tones in the therapist's voice (who is also middle-aged), was perhaps a contributor to the unsatisfactory conclusion of this interchange. The therapist let his feelings show through in an untoward manner. The therapist here should immediately have picked up and used the patient's name for the man he was replacing, and he should have noted his own sympathy for the older man and a twinge of animosity toward the patient. He should have not allowed his feelings to contaminate the interview.

A therapist rarely should decline to explore a subject or event that a patient wishes to discuss. Such a refusal may cause the patient to feel that the topic or event is dangerous, or repulsive, or in some other way unacceptable. In other cases he may feel that the therapist feels it is irrelevant to spend time on something which the patient nevertheless finds troublesome. When this kind of topic is broached by the patient the therapist at times may say, "Since this is important to you, we shall talk about it." At other times the therapist may say,

"In this room we can talk about any subject or anything that has happened in your life. When we've looked at it thoroughly, we can decide how important it really is." When a therapist feels that a patient is apprehensive about his reaction to a subject the therapist occasionally may add, "Do you fear that if everything in your life is brought out into the open, I'll eventually become discouraged with you as a patient or reject you as a person? That doesn't happen here. Our job is to examine all your life, not just those parts of it that you feel are presentable."

Investigation of the patient's daydreams, or fantasies, is sometimes useful, but the interpersonal purposes of this should be kept constantly in mind and at times should be defined to the patient. "Everyone daydreams a great deal, all his life. By talking about them we may find out a good deal about your hopes and fears, your views of yourself and what you feel is missing, or excessive, in you and your life. It makes no difference whether the daydream is practical or impractical, or could possibly be realized one day or not; daydreams can sometimes tell us much about a person's emotional inner life and his day-to-day relationships with people."

However, discussion of daydreams should occupy only a small part of the total time of a course of therapy and it should always be tied to actual events and relationships in the patient's life. "Let us examine your daydream of being a glamorous, famous, wealthy pop star in terms of what would happen to your relationships with your parents and friends if that were to occur." "If these daydreams of becoming president of the company and making it even more successful than it is were to come true, what effects would such things have on your relationships with your wife and your teenage children?" "If you were actually to die in the tragic way you daydream about, what would the close people in your life feel? What would be the effects on them?" If daydreams are not tied in with the patient's ongoing and past life, but are allowed to acquire an independent sphere of their own, and much time is spent talking about them, they cast a shadow of unreality over therapy.

To summarize, daydreams may be informative about the patient's private, or inner, emotional life, but they should be extrapolated into useful data for the therapeutic goal, which is to help the patient achieve new levels of emotional health and in living with people in his day-to-day life. In Chapter 8 we shall deal with the topic of dreams which occur during sleep.

4 Emotional Well-Being and Well-Being Operations

A person who has emotional well-being is free of anxiety, guilt, depression, self-loathing, and other forms of emotional pain. As a result he can adjust well both in the close and the broader relationships of his life; he or she does well in his family life and in his social, economic, and cultural activities in the community.

Each person throughout his life seeks sound levels of emotional well-being; he wants to be free of emotional distress and unsatisfying or conflict-ridden relationships with people. No one achieves this goal completely. No environment is ever static and new situations arise to create small or large problems that should be resolved as smoothly and quickly as possible. Also, every person has some emotional liabilities and personality shortcomings. Meeting and resolving emotional problems is a never-ending process.

The ways in which a person seeks these goals are called well-being operations. A healthy person has an ample repertory of well-being operations and a badly adjusted person uses defective ones or lacks them altogether. In this chapter we shall discuss what well-being operations are and how they function in health, illness, and psychotherapy.

The Role of Well-Being Operations in Daily Life

A well-being operation is an interpersonal activity by which an individual reduces emotional pain; he or she can then relate better to others. A person may or may not be aware of his ways of achieving emotional and interpersonal ease; he may carry them out without understanding them or even being aware of them. However, many people are aware of the ways they do these things and can talk clearly about them.

A well-being operation may be healthy or unhealthy in all situations in which it occurs, or it may be healthy in some situations and unhealthy in others. For example, a child who is censured harshly by her mother for something she has done may in turn severely reprimand her doll; in this case the well-being operation is healthy. In contrast, if an adult who is bawled out by his work supervisor for negligence then does the same thing with the people under him, who have not been negligent, he is carrying out an unhealthy well-being operation. In both cases the individual has reduced his own emotional discomfort, which is the object of a well-being operation, but the child has acted in a healthy way and the adult has not.

Both healthy and unhealthy well-being operations decrease emotional pain, but an unhealthy one distorts or contaminates some facet of the individual's interpersonal life. This is illustrated in the case of the adult cited above. Moreover, in some instances an unhealthy well-being operation causes a marked emotional discomfort to be replaced by a less severe one, and in the process some limitation or defect is introduced into the patient's life. The adult described above is relieved of feelings of worthlessness and personal inadequacy caused by his supervisor's criticism, but he has alienated his work force, which may cause him many problems in the future. Put another way, it is a sick solution.

It should be stressed that every well-being operation by definition involves things that go on between two or more people. It is observable. The child cited above can be seen and heard as she chastises her doll and the man's activities are seen and heard by a number of involved people. A well-being operation is not an inner unobservable, and therefore hypothetical, process, which can never be clearly demonstrated and laid open for objective study.

Healthy Well-Being Operations

Perceptive Inattention

In the well-being operation of perceptive inattention a person does not perceive various things that are going on in his environment. At any moment each individual perceives only a small part of what is occurring in his surroundings and that part is selected according to his emotional and intellectual needs at the time. Perceptive inattention is necessary for successful living; without it life would be overwhelmingly complex and disorganized.

For example, a person who is reading this book is attentive to what he is reading and is not perceiving, or is perceiving only to a limited extent, what his or her roommate is discussing on a telephone a short distance away. Such perceptive inattention is mandatory if he or she is to understand what he reads. Clear perception of the telephone conversation would make understanding the book difficult or impossible. In a general way the reader may be aware of the nearby conversation, but it is meaningless to him. This is a healthy example of perceptive inattention in its most simple form.

Let us alter the situation and assume that the reader is a woman and that her fiancé enters the room. She lowers the book and the two of them discuss their plans to go to a basketball game that night. They decide that an hour before the game begins the fiancé will drop by the apartment of another woman and ask her to accompany them to the game. In this event the woman does not perceive that while they were discussing their plans to go to the game her fiancé was bored and listless, but that when the other woman was mentioned he became alert. These things were excluded from her awareness by perceptive inattention; it would have been painful for her to be aware of her fiancé's lack of interest in going with her alone and his eager interest in the woman who was to accompany them. In this instance perceptive inattention is an unhealthy well-being operation because it excludes from this woman's realm of perceived experience information that it would be much better for her to have.

This unhealthy perceptive inattention operation has had a small advantage and a large disadvantage for the woman. The small advantage is that she has been spared the pain of becoming aware of her fiancé's waning interest in her and the substitution of the other woman in her place. The disadvantage is that she does not have the kind of informed experience she needs to make the best possible adjustment in a difficult situation. If she is four months pregnant by her fiancé the disadvantage is much greater.

The pressing question now is, how easily can this woman cease to perceptively inattend bodies of experience that she must have to address this problem in the best possible way.

Let us assume that when the fiancé leaves the apartment to pick up the other woman, her roommate, who observed what happened, says, "Did you notice anything wrong in Tony's reactions to your plans for this evening? He seemed a lot more interested in going to the game after you decided to take Susan along." If the involved woman for any reason casts this observation aside she is acting unhealthily. If on the contrary she lays her book down and says, "If you think there's something going on that I haven't seen and ought to know about, tell me. It will be rough on me, but I can't do whatever's needed unless I know what the situation is," she is taking a healthy step to solve her problem. She does it by ceasing to use perceptive inattention as a sick well-being operation.

Perceptive inattention can occur only in the present. A person cannot fail to perceive something that happened in the past. When an individual has excluded some experience by perceptive inattention it is not part of his fund of perceived, assimilated experience and is not available to him in meeting and solving his problems.

Sublimation

In the well-being operation of sublimation a person achieves socially acceptable expressions of emotional forces that would harm his relationships with people if he or she expressed them directly. For example, aggressive, hostile feelings may be expressed in competitive sports such as football and hockey. Sexual urges may be released by communicating with people in esthetic pursuits such as music and painting. Sculpting and playing the drums sublimate both aggressive and sexual-esthetic drives. In many types of altruistic activities people attenuate sexual feelings by affectionate work to help others.

In some cases it is easy to trace strong feelings through to their sublimated expressions; for example, a person who beats a rug on a clothesline or does some other form of vigorous work to avoid an angry argument with his or her spouse, or an individual who seizes golf clubs and goes to a driving range after an exasperating day at work. In many other instances the connection between a strong emotion and its sublimated expression is conjectural.

Sublimation is usually a healthy well-being operation. It helps people to be comfortable in many situations in day-to-day life. However, in some cases it is unhealthy. An individual who speeds on city streets to give release to angry feelings and a person who throws expensive dinner plates against a wall to avoid a brawl with his or her marital partner are sublimating in self-defeating, unhealthy ways.

Identification

A person forms many of the features of his personality in the contexts of his interactions with people in his day-to-day environment, especially during childhood and the first years of adolescence. A healthy personality depends on identifications with persons who are meeting their daily problems in sound ways; an unhealthy identification occurs in the contexts of troubled relationships. Thus a boy who identifies with (i.e., absorbs or takes on the characteristics of) a brutal, violent father is forming an unhealthy identification, and a girl who absorbs the qualities of an affectionate, well-adjusted mother is making a healthy one. Every growing child and adolescent takes on features of both his parents as a rule and, to a lesser extent, those of close neighbors and other long-term companions. To some extent he also is influenced by what he experiences while watching television, seeing videos, and reading. No one is a carbon copy of some other person, no matter how massive that person's influence has been.

A psychotherapist may at times be concerned with identification as a well-being operation; in this capacity identification may obscure many forms of emotional discomfort and disturbance. It is as if the patient were saying, "What I am doing is sound and good because it's what the important persons in my life did." Thus the boy who identifies with a brutal, violent father in effect says, "Only by fighting and keeping everyone off balance can you hold your own and prevent them from dominating you."

An identification (like a personality) is similar to a tree; some of its roots are large and some are small, some are strong and some are weak, some are sound and some are diseased, but they all contribute to the tree.

Compensatory Reactions

A good example of a compensatory well-being operation is seen in the surgeon described in the opening part of Chapter 2. He was reared by a harsh, unaffectionate, belittling father and an emotionally indifferent mother and emerged into late adolescence and early adulthood with gnawing fears about his worth as a person. In reaction to these fears he attempted to compensate by becoming an achieving, valued member of society. However, in doing so he put himself on a treadmill to prove constantly to himself and to others that he was not the depreciated person his upbringing had led him to fear he was. When we met him, he had decompensated because of the consequences of an error in his professional practice.

A compensation reaction frequently is a healthy well-being operation in response to unhealthy emotional forces. Our surgeon, instead of developing a constructive well-being operation, might have made an unhealthy adjustment to his unperceived fears. In such a case he might have become an alcoholic who sought to blur his inner distresses by drinking or a chronic philanderer who by many brief sexual adventures sought endlessly to reassure himself that he was a desired, valued, attractive person.

Other Healthy Well-Being Operations

In a book on psychotherapy it would be inappropriate to go further in our discussion of the various kinds of healthy well-being operations, but the coverage that has been given indicates that a therapist must be interested in many of the healthy, as well as unhealthy, well-being operations in each of his patients. This is because healthy well-being operations sometimes break down and cause problems in living. Our surgeon, once more, is a good example of this.

Unhealthy Well-Being Operations

In an unhealthy well-being operation a person reduces emotional pain and increases his comfort at a certain cost. This cost may consist of a limitation or defect in his interpersonal capacities or a new emotional discomfort that is more tolerable than the original one. For example, a person who withdraws from contacts with others because he finds interpersonal relationships painful is more at ease; but his life has become barren and uncomfortable; loneliness may afflict him. In a similar way, an individual who resolves large amounts of anxiety by developing compulsions and obsessions is freed from much of his anxiousness but must cope with repetitive acts and thoughts that may vary from minor annoyances to social incapacitations.

Unhealthy well-being operations are commonly encountered in psychotherapy; in many cases they are the main problem for which the patient is seeking help. The patient who wants help for his withdrawal from people wants to be more comfortable with them, and the obsessive-compulsive patient wants to be rid of his repetitive thoughts and acts. Each patient wants a better adjustment in life and as comfortable an existence as he can achieve.

We shall consider a few of the common unhealthy well-being operations.

Withdrawal from People

Withdrawal from people may vary in degree from moderate shyness to the profound retreat from others, which is labeled a schizoid personality disorder. Withdrawal from people is caused by prolonged painful trauma in close relationships during childhood and the first years of adolescence. Instead of receiving affection and esteem as a person, the individual who withdraws experienced coldness, rejection, and depreciation. To him closeness with others seems a painful prison rather than a healthy way of life. By withdrawal he diminishes the possibilities of pain, which others might inflict on him and in this sense he gains something; however, his withdrawal may rob him of the satisfactions of marriage, stimulating relationships with children, gratifying teamwork with co-workers, and many other kinds of social rewards. Moreover, the relief obtained by diminished contacts with people is only partial because the withdrawn individual continues to suffer in the unavoidable interactions that economic life and day-to-day necessities require.

The person whose life is dominated by the unhealthy well-being operation of withdrawal lacks much information that can be acquired and constantly updated only in brisk associations with others. He may be unaware of many things that affect him as a member of a work force, as a member of his community, and as a participant in inescapable social and economic activities. He becomes out of touch with what people around him are feeling, thinking, and doing about both small and large things. He tends to be bypassed or to be left in some awkward corner of the social world. People may at times be jolted by things such an individual says and does because of his defective awareness of his milieu.

Regression

In the unhealthy well-being operation of regression a person diminishes the pain of an interpersonal situation by retreating into a role that is less mature than expected for one of his or her age or by retiring into a more dependent status than he formerly had. For example, a 5-year-old child may become anxious about his place in his parents' affection when a sibling is born and, competing with the newborn child, regresses in speech, toilet training, and eating habits. An adult may regress into sickness with its involved dependency on others; the symptoms of his regression may cluster around an emotional or physical difficulty, which he already had but which now becomes worse. In other cases the entire clinical picture is new. Thus a person who finds it difficult to meet the everyday problems of marriage and parenthood may descend into semi-invalidism based on muscular pains and weakness. This may happen not only when a minor myositis or bursitis preceded the incapacitating syndrome, but also when the whole group of shoulder and arm symptoms is new. The same thing may happen to a person who is having difficulties in a work situation; work related symptoms are notoriously more difficult to resolve if the symptoms take the individual out of disagreeable work and, by financial compensation, make him independent of it.

Though in regression a person's total life adjustment suffers he has decreased the interpersonal and physical stresses of a situation that was problematic for him. His well-being operation takes him out of the difficult situation or eliminates the necessity of dealing with home-based problems.

Denial

In some cases a person denies the existence of painful circumstances. This, for example, may occur in the parents of mentally retarded children. They may say that their children "will grow out of it" or "can't get along in the rough and tumble of today's schools." Such denials may continue until adolescence brings problems such as the sexual exploitation of girls or the economic exploitation of both sexes, aggravated by fitful adolescent rebellion; such difficulties make at least partial acceptance of the situation imperative. These parents avoid the pain of recognizing their children's limitations but do so at the cost of depriving them of the best possible up-bringing and education, which would ease the later lives of both the children and themselves.

In a similar way people may deny the presence of severe marital incompatibilities, obvious infidelities by spouses, obvious drug addiction or alcohol abuse, gross exploitation in jobs, and many other problems. By denial, limited emotional peace is secured at the expense of marked difficulties in the short or long run. In some instances denials last for decades or a lifetime as persons or families lurch from one difficulty or crisis to the next. An entrenched well-being operation of denial may be difficult to address in therapy, and in some instances, unless the therapist is sure that something better can be substituted in its place, it is best to leave it alone. Such decisions require astute clinical judgment and a comprehensive evaluation of the patient and his interpersonal world.

Obsessive and Compulsive Thoughts and Acts

In this group of unhealthy well-being operations a person decreases emotional suffering at the cost of developing repetitive thoughts and acts. These may vary from annoyances, such as double checking all gas outlets, faucets, and electrical switches before leaving the house, to incapacitating rituals, such as daylong washing of the hands and the bathroom.

There is a magical quality in obsessive-compulsive well-being operations. Magic may be sympathetic or imitative, or a combination of the two. In sympathetic magic a person attempts to control a situation (in this case psychological turmoil) by thinking or doing things that are similar in some way to the inner distress, and in imitative magic an individual attempts the same thing by performing in his thoughts and acts essential features of the causative force. For example, painful sexual thoughts such as masturbatory guilt or barely perceived homosexual urges may be symbolically washed away by repetitive cleansing of the hands and body. Aggressive thoughts and impulses may be expressed in a necessity to stamp on each dividing mark in a sidewalk or to strike each post in a fence or grating. Elaborate counting rituals, such as counting each step as a door is approached or a corridor is traversed and beginning or ending such a process with the right or left foot, are common. In all these cases a more comfortable emotional state is achieved at the expense of inconvenience or outright social incapacitation. Repetitive thoughts may serve a similar function. One of our patients who was much disturbed by religious doubts developed an obsessive quandry about whether or not God was baldheaded. By this ever-circling thought she was freed from what was for her a much more threatening thought, whether or not God existed.

The steps by which obsessive-compulsive well-being operations develop can at times be directly observed. This is illustrated in the case of a 13-year-old patient of ours. This boy ejaculated onto his undershirt while masturbating in the bathroom. He washed these marks from his undershirt and then washed his hands. During the next 48 hours he developed an elaborate cleaning ritual in which he washed his hands, arms, and body and scrubbed the bathroom walls, fixtures, and floor; these acts lasted all day long and at times far into the night. When we saw him shortly after this he was able to give a step-by-step account of the evolution of his compulsions and the accompanying obsessions of physical and moral dirtiness. He felt he was "washing away the filth" of his masturbation. In most cases a therapist sees an obsessive-compulsive patient after his symptoms have been present for weeks or months and he can no longer recall the steps by which they developed.

Other Unhealthy Well-Being Operations

There are many other types of unhealthy well-being operations. In their totality they cause many of the psychiatric problems, both large and small, that therapists encounter.

Well-Being Operations Encountered in Problem-Oriented Psychotherapy

When a person in psychotherapy has a rising level of anxiety, guilt, self-loathing, shame, or some other distress in reaction to a painful topic he is discussing, he may, in ways he does not perceive, resort to a well-being operation to push that topic aside. In Chapter 3 a patient used *irrelevant verbosity* in this way; she deviated into rapid, forced talking about the business career of an acquaintance to avoid the nearer subject of marital infidelity. The patient who uses irrelevant verbosity to veer away from a distressing topic in treatment often does the same thing in his home, workplace, and social environments. If he can make progress in recognizing and abandoning this unhealthy well-being operation in therapy and become clearly aware of its roots and ramifications, he can begin to do the same thing in many other settings. He gets rid of the verbal smoke screens which have long hampered him.

Blanket Agreement

Complete unhesitating agreement with something the therapist says tends to stifle further discussion of the subject.

Therapist: When Dusty said that you must have felt desolate and abandoned.

Patient: Yes, I did.

Therapist: Can you tell me more about what you felt and what thoughts you had at that point?

Patient: You seem to have summed it up pretty well.

Therapist: Had you felt such desolation with him before?

Patient: At times.

Therapist: And abandoned?

Patient: Yes.

Where does a therapist go at this point? The patient has shut off further exploration of this event by blanket agreement with the therapist. The proper step for the therapist now (and he should not fall into the trap of labeling such parroting of his words as "insight") is to concentrate on the patient's well-being operation. For the time being this is more important than examination of what happened in this incident.

Therapist: Would it be fair to say that by immediate entire agreement with me you shut off further exploration of this painful episode in your relationship with Dusty?

Patient: Huh?

Therapist: When you agreed so promptly and fully with what I said—that you felt desolate and abandoned—you left us little more to talk about regarding this event.

Patient: I guess so.

Therapist: Do you tend to do the same thing when you're talking with other people?

Patient: Edith says she can never get a rise out of me, even when she wants to.

Therapist: Does she like this aspect of you?

Patient: I guess not. Edith says it's like reaching out to grab me and I'm not there. My brother says that sometimes talking with me is like shadow boxing.

As we have previously noted, the only interpersonal relationship in the patient's life that is available for direct scrutiny is the one he has with the therapist. That relationship often is a fruitful area for exploration. Problem-oriented psychotherapy does not view this as a form of transference of feelings and thoughts. A patient does not transfer feelings and thoughts from other areas of his life into his relationship with the therapist; he merely continues to employ with the therapist the same characteristic well-being operations, both sick and healthy (as well as his other interpersonal ways of relating), that he utilizes in all other relationships. Problem-oriented psychotherapy also does not accept the idea that in dealing with these things a patient "works through" what he "transfers" and in doing so relives old relationships and solves emotional problems that were not resolved in them.

No one ever relives anything. Each relationship in a person's life is a new one and each day is unlike any preceding one. Personality change occurs by developing new ways of living, not by re-experiencing events in relationships that existed in the past. This subject is more extensively considered in Chapter 7.

Attacks on the Therapist

Another type of unhealthy well-being operation in psychotherapy is attacking the therapist.

Therapist: Do you feel that your competitive attitudes and acts at work and elsewhere are in the end self-defeating?
Patient: Of course, and I've known that for years. I didn't enter therapy to hear things like that. You retail a lot of expensive platitudes, don't you?
Therapist: Does it help you to blow off steam in this way?
Patient: No. Incidentally, do I get a refund on all the time that we waste here?

Therapist: Do you often use an attack, both here and elsewhere, to avoid talking about a painful topic—to block
awareness of some uncomfortable aspect of how you get
along with people?

Erotic Overtures

An erotic overture to the therapist is one of various well-
being operations that attempt to turn the therapeutic situation into a social one. Patients of both sexes may do this. An
experienced psychotherapist whom we knew used to say to
patients at such a point, "What you are suggesting might be
fun, but we have important work to do." He could combine
these words with just the right voice tones and verbal emphases to reject the patient's overture without rejecting the
patient. At such a juncture the therapist can broaden the
discussion by exploring whether or not the patient characteristically tries to shunt aside threatening things in interpersonal relationships by injecting erotic notes into them. "When
you feel your job is threatened, or that someone is going to
refuse to do something that is important for you, or that
you're not going to get a grade you feel you must have in your
university course, do you tend to insert a sexy note into the
proceedings?" "Is this one of the ways in which you react in
many kinds of person-to-person stresses? When the crunch is
on do you sometimes find yourself flirting?"

Problem-oriented psychotherapy does not accept the concept that an erotic move by a patient represents feelings origi-
nally directed at a parent and that the patient is attempting to
relive and resolve an erotic relationship from that time that
ended traumatically. Understanding and handling sexual
overtures, and in the process turning them into useful ave-
nues of therapy, should occupy a special place in the training
of psychotherapists.

This general subject is covered in more detail in Chapter 7.

Praising the Therapist

ı nıs is a well-being operation that occasionally is encountered in psychotherapy.

Therapist: So far we have not talked much about your marriage.

Patient: I'm feeling so much better and my ways of handling things have improved so much that I don't think that's going to be necessary. You've done a lot for me. People comment on it. They say I'm a different person. I guess I'm a pretty good advertisement for you.

Therapist: Does your wife share these views?

Patient: She's your number one fan.

The patient here is attempting to avoid discussion of his marriage by flattering the therapist. The therapist should avoid the attractive trap of misinterpreting this as progress.

Other kinds of undesirable well-being operations occur in psychotherapy; sometimes more than one of them are going on at the same time. In other instances they alternate as the patient tries to shunt the interview away from emotionally painful material. In many cases a large part of psychotherapy is spent in working on these problems.

Other Aspects of Managing Well-Being Operations

A therapist should not attempt to modify or remove an unhealthy well-being operation unless he feels he can offer a healthier way of interacting in its place. This should occur only when the patient has the capacity to incorporate it into his day-to-day living.

The following dialogue, which would be longer and more detailed in ongoing therapy, illustrates this principle. The patient has a phobia of small, enclosed places—a claustrophobia.

Patient: On Thursday I got on the elevator and went from the ground floor to our offices on the fifth floor. That's the first time I've done that in a long time. I'm improving.

Therapist: Was it comfortable?

Patient: I was edgy, but that's progress for me.

Therapist: Were you alone or was someone with you?

Patient: Phil Jaffe was with me.

Therapist: Who is he?

Patient: He's a customer. He buys a lot from us.

Therapist: How did you and Phil Jaffe happen to be going up to your office?

Patient: I had a business lunch with him and afterward he wanted to see the designs of our new line of overhead transfer belts. He's thinking of installing them in his warehouse.

Therapist: When you set up this business lunch did you anticipate that he'd be going to your office afterward?

Patient: No, I thought I'd just get my pitch in sometime during lunch and then he'd think it over, but he liked the idea and wanted to move right along with it.

Therapist: How did you feel as you approached the elevator?

Patient: Pretty tense, I guess.

Therapist: Looking back at it, would you have used the elevator, or would you have walked up, if Phil Jaffe hadn't been with you?

Patient: I probably would have chickened out and walked up.

Therapist: Do you feel at times that you have to present evidence to me of progress in this treatment even if you have to force it a little? (*The therapist's voice tones and a slight smile make this an invitation to talk and not an accusation.*)

Patient: (Laughs uneasily) My wife says I do it with her. She says she can't see many signs of progress.

Therapist: Does anyone else say that?

Patient: My partner keeps asking if I can now do this or that, especially regarding small conference rooms and the kinds of cubbyholes that seem everywhere in our line of business. He says that when I can sit down in one of those dictating booths for half an hour he'll feel that I've accomplished something.

Therapist: Are you able to manage a dictating booth even for a short time now?

Patient: Not yet.

Therapist: Would it be correct to say that you feel a need to reassure me that you're making progress, even if you have to stretch it a good deal?

Patient: I guess so.

Therapist: Do you feel this same kind of need to keep people satisfied in your relationships in general? In other words, do you work pretty hard to prevent others from becoming dissatisfied, or frankly irritated, with you?

Patient: My wife says I do. She calls it "doormatting."

Therapist: Can you give me an example of what she calls "doormatting"?

Patient: When our kids have trouble with the kids next door she's always the one who ends up talking to their parents about it. She says I'm so anxious to please everybody that I can't straighten out things like that.

Therapist: Let your imagination freewheel for a minute. What do you think might happen if you were more assertive with the neighbors when these problems come up?

Patient: Well, they might get upset with me.

Therapist: Upset?

Patient: Angry. Get mad at me.

Therapist: And then what would happen?

Patient: They might not want to have anything more to do with me.

Therapist: Do they do that with your wife when she has to settle something with them?

Patient: No.

Therapist: How do they treat her?

Patient: All right. I guess they respect her more than they do me. When something goes wrong they blow off steam at me. They don't do that with her.

Therapist: Does the same general sort of of thing happen when you, as a couple, have any other kind of problem with people?

Patient: Yes, Caroline says I go "doormatting" all over the place and that if I stuck up for myself people would listen to me more.

Therapist: And does she add that the rejection you fear if you were assertive would rarely materialize? In fact, that things would be better afterward between you and people?

Patient: She says that people don't hold grudges about little things like that.

Therapist: Going back to your need to reassure me that you're making progress in treatment, what do you think would happen if you didn't do that?

Patient: I should think you'd get pretty sick and tired of seeing me.

Therapist: In other words, reject you, perhaps terminate treatment.

Patient: Something like that.

Therapist: I think we've outlined a central problem here, one that causes you a good deal of inner turmoil at home, at work, in social groups, and even in your treatment with me. There are healthier ways of dealing with people than "doormatting," and all the feelings you bottle up in the process would not rumble around inside you and fuel your fear of small places. Being reasonably assertive—sticking up for yourself—will usually bring you respect and acceptance, not rejection.

The therapist here has (1) identified an unhealthy well-being operation of the patient ("doormatting") and (2) has offered a healthier mode of living (reasonable assertiveness) to take its place. He thus has adhered to the principle of problem-oriented psychotherapy that an unhealthy well-being operation should not be removed until the therapist has a better way of living to put in its place and is sure, moreover, that the patient is ready to accept this new way and act on it.

The Third-Party Technique

In this procedure the therapist in essence says, "It's difficult for you to talk about this. Let's approach it from a different angle. Say that someone, whom we shall call John Miller, and who is about your age and matches you in other ways, finds himself doing . . ." The therapist then sketches the patient's problems in terms of this hypothetical person, John Miller. For example, the therapist might continue, "John Miller finds himself periodically in conflict with people who are in authority over him, especially older people such as parents, work supervisors, and leaders in social groups. In addition to resentment and resistance toward them, what other feelings do you think he might have?" In some cases a patient talks easily about his problems (and knows he is talking about them) in this way. The simple substitution of *he* for *I* smoothes the way.

In another form of the third-party technique an imaginary observer is introduced into one of the patient's interpersonal situations. Thus the therapist says, "I wonder what an outsider who was watching this event would have said and thought about it. Let's consider it from this angle. When Al told you he was leaving you for good what would this observer have said about your reaction?"

The third-party technique, adjusted to their age level, is particularly useful in working with children. With children this is more often a technique for giving information than for getting it. "You know, I once had a patient whose problems were exactly like yours. His name was Jimmy Green and he was . . ." It is best always to employ the same name, such as Jimmy Green or Joannie Green, because children sometimes ask weeks or months later what was the name of that other boy or girl who had troubles just like his, and if the therapist does not use the same name with all patients, he may be in a difficult position. We feel that the use of such a hypothetical patient with children is clinically honest since Jimmy or Joannie Green is a composite of other patients whom the therapist has seen and read about.

As mentioned briefly in Chapter 1 in another context, work on a well-being operation should begin with interpersonal events and relationships in the patient's present or recent past and then proceed into earlier periods. For example, the difficulties of the last patient in the dialogue above (the phobic patient) are addressed in terms of things that are going on in his present work situation and other current settings. The same problems can then be examined in past experiences at college; during adolescence with persons of both sexes; and with his mother, father, and siblings in both early and later childhood. These early relationships, especially with parents, as a rule constitute the most important area, but to begin with them often is upsetting and a therapeutic mistake. Most patients find this a more comfortable and productive way to proceed in discussing anxiety-laden aspects of their lives.

The therapist and the patient examine what the patient is doing, and is going to do, with his new insights and personality capacities in his day-to-day life. New ways of living may create problems of their own and solutions must be found for them. For example, when a markedly passive individual becomes more comfortable with assertiveness and is increasingly aggressive, can his spouse accept him as someone who can no longer be taken for granted or even dominated? When an adolescent or a young adult, who has been overprotected by engulfing parents, moves toward independent action, are his parents able to accept this or do they see it as a rejection of themselves and react accordingly? When a withdrawn adolescent or young adult begins to move into wider interpersonal circles and to form close ties with persons of the opposite sex, does he or she know how to handle the many small and large problems involved? Does he or she really know what to do on a date and what other people expect of him in many kinds of events that are new to him? How much help, sometimes in the nature of practical advice and guidance, do various kinds of patients need in these areas? Some patients need little such help or none at all, but others need varying amounts of it if they are to avoid pitfalls and discouraging interpersonal failures.

Insight is not enough. It must be firmly incorporated into what the patient feels, thinks, and does in all facets of his life, both during the time he is in treatment and in the long periods that stretch out beyond that.

What Is a Personality?

A personality consists of all the characteristic ways in which an individual interacts with others, and his feelings, thoughts, and actions in those situations. His well-being operations, both healthy and unhealthy, constitute a significant segment of his personality.

This is illustrated in the following example. If asked to sketch the personality of a friend, a person might say that, among many other things, he (1) gets along well with people but is somewhat shy and awkward with people whom he does not know well, (2) can be affectionate, but only after he has known a person for a long time and when that person has clearly indicated that he or she likes him, (3) learns new things quickly and is able to apply what he has learned but hesitates to do so unless he is in a circle of people by whom he feels accepted, (4) tends to withdraw from others into reading, listening to music, and watching television and videos when friction occurs in his interpersonal life and (5) has headaches and gastrointestinal upsets when he must persist in stressful situations. As indicated, this person has many other characteristics, but the ones we have listed are sufficient to illustrate what we mean by a personality. Some of these five features are well-being operations.

All these things can be seen and heard in talking with this individual, in observing him, in talking with others about him, and in examining other data relevant to his current and past life. It is not composed of unobservable, and therefore unverifiable, abstractions that lie beyond the limits of scientific investigation and thinking.

An individual's characteristic ways of interacting with people are molded by his relationships with them. Early close relationships, writing on a blank or nearly blank slate, are most important in this respect, but a personality never becomes a fixed, rigid thing. The associations a person has with others all his life, and the many social and economic forces that have impacts on him, continue to modify him. The person sketched immediately above, for example, was reared by a controlling but affectionate mother and a father who was passive and retiring but fond of him. Later events and relationships have modified him. His skill as a computer programmer in a new field with a fresh generation of computers has given him prestige among his peers and superiors, and has been constructive; a rebuff in his first passionate relationship with a woman has been a negative factor. What he will be like twenty or forty years in the future can be speculated upon only in the broadest way. It is this malleability of personality structures that in the final analysis makes psychotherapy possible.

In our opinion even when the human genome has in the distant future been fully worked out and its influence on personality is understood, the things that occur after birth will be more important than those that occur before it in determining an individual's personality.

5 Making and Testing Tentative Formulations

Verification is a basic process in problem-oriented psychotherapy; in it the therapist and the patient reach a conclusion about some aspect of the patient's way of living that they previously have formulated tentatively. For example, after examining with the patient many events and relationships in his life the therapist advances the tentative formulation that the patient tends to withdraw emotionally from each situation in which tension occurs. This withdrawal prevents him from ever resolving any interpersonal problem. Then in a joint venture of shared involvement they look at many things that go on, and have gone on, in his life to see if this tentative formulation is valid. In this process the tentative formulation may have to be modified or even abandoned. Regardless of the outcome much has been learned about the patient's feelings, thoughts, and interpersonal patterns, and often the therapist and he are then able to put forth a new formulation that undergoes the same process. Psychotherapy moves from one such formulation to another and in the end these formulations join together to give a broad view of the kind of person the patient is and how he came to be that way.

All psychotherapeutic formulations are at first tentative. Every experienced therapist can recall many patients about whom he felt he had reached firm conclusions only to find that they had to be revised as he learned more about the patient. The term tentative formulation merely summarizes a general truth.

The broaching of a tentative formulation and its verification are illustrated in the following abridged patient–therapist dialogue. The patient is a 33-year-old physician.

Therapist: Dr. Sachs, as we have been discussing what goes on between you and other people both now and in the past, I have gradually been forming an idea about your relationships with them. Any coldness or indifference in a person with whom you are beginning to get close causes you to back off. You attenuate the relationship or abandon it altogether. Perhaps we can explore this to see if it is actually so. We are interested not only in whether you do this but also why. (*The therapist has here set forth a tentative formulation and has set the stage for its verification.*)

Patient: Well, I guess that's the way it is in my relationships with women. If a girl turns me down for a date, no matter what she says in doing so, it's the last time I call her.

Therapist: Did the same thing go on earlier in your life, say when you were in medical school?

Patient: I was a loner. I always needed a strong green light from people, and people usually don't go around giving strong green lights. I know it's a little unreasonable on my part, but if I don't get that kind of encouragement I figure the situation is not for me.

Therapist: What about other areas of your life?

Patient: At the club I'm mainly a golfer. If a couple of people are teeing off and ask me to go around with them I do, but

I never take the initiative in such things. I never ask if I can join them.

Therapist: For fear they might say no?

Patient: I guess so.

Therapist: Does the same thing happen in your relationships with patients?

Patient: Not really. If a patient is uncooperative or irritable I figure it's his illness that's making him that way, and so I get along with patients pretty well. Even the argumentative ones like me. The girls at the clinic comment on it. An internist like me spends half his time taking care of middle-aged and elderly people with heart disease, hypertension, diabetes, arthritis, and such problems; people with chronic illnesses tend to get upset with their doctors once in a while. That sort of thing doesn't bother me. I even go so far as to call them on the phone to find out why they missed appointments. I'm the same way with patients of all ages. With patients I don't need a green light. It's the other way around.

Therapist: How do you *feel* about working with resistant patients?

Patient: I enjoy it. The girls at the clinic say I'm married to the place and that the patients are my family. I meet them more than halfway. My hours are always full. I joke with the cantankerous ones. I say things like, "Well, Mrs. Jones, what are you going to give me hell about today?" and we both laugh.

Therapist: Then in this area of your life coldness from people doesn't seem to cause you to withdraw.

Patient: I wouldn't be much of a doctor if it did.

Therapist: It may be more important than that. It's healthy in a much broader sense. If we can discover why this segment of your life is different for you we perhaps can make progress in the areas in which you don't have the same capacity.

The therapist has had to modify his original formulation and in doing so a new channel for psychotherapy has been opened.

Special Aspects of Verifying Formulations

When he makes a tentative formulation the therapist should mobilize as little emotional discomfort in the patient as possible for, as we saw in Chapter 3, feelings of anxiety, guilt, personal worthlessness, and other forms of emotional distress make exploration of a subject difficult.

This is particularly so in the cases of withdrawn patients. Such a person has long felt that people are insensitive to his needs and that interpersonal closeness is a prison, not an opportunity. If the therapist's tentative formulation with this kind of patient is inaccurate the patient may feel it as a crude probing of a wound. He retreats, injured and puzzled that this has occurred in a relationship that is supposed to be helping him. In general, therefore, a tentative interpretation should be presented to a markedly withdrawn person only when the evidence for its validity is so strong that it has almost ceased to be tentative. By that time the patient has gradually accepted so much of it that the therapist's task consists mainly in putting into clear, concise language what the patient and he have long been talking about.

Verification is a process that corrects misverifications that occurred earlier in a patient's life. For example, the unduly aggressive person during childhood and adolescence often formed a misverification that he could hold his own with other people only by constantly attacking them and keeping them on the defensive. Out of conflicts with harsh or indifferent parents, at times coupled with abrasive rivalry with siblings and others, he developed this feeling. Each individual's imbedded patterns of feeling, thinking, and interacting with others are products of his life situations. They seem reasonable to him; they seem to be the only way of living. The passive person's life experiences have led him, frequently in ways he can only dimly perceive, to feel that deferring to others and ingratiating himself with them is the best way to relate to them. Psychotherapeutic verification is a healing process made necessary by prior misverifications.

There are no essential differences between the ways in which people get sick and the ways by which they can be helped to get well. Unhealthy misverifications cause personality illness and healthy verifications aid people to adjust more comfortably and effectively. In this process much that was not perceived becomes perceived; much that lay in the patient's realm of unawareness moves into the region of awareness. Nonperception is replaced by emotional and intellectual awareness in a gradual process of accretion and assimilation.

A psychotic patient has suffered severe losses in his capacity for verification; he has withdrawn both from people and the material world about him to such an extent that he is unable to have the healing, sound relationships that could help him. In the consequent vacuum the schizophrenic develops hallucinatory and delusional experiences. A severely depressed patient is so weighed down by a self-deprecatory view of himself and a hopeless outlook on the world (and that world includes the therapist) that a similar dearth of ongoing helpful experience, and the capacity for it, exists. The same problems are present in the manic patient with his helter-skelter mental and physical excitement and his inability to concentrate on anything for more than a minute or two. The paranoid patient fears that malicious people are ubiquitously about him. Psychotherapy alone is hence rarely successful with psychotic patients and antipsychotic medication in a therapeutic environment must be employed.

The following patient–therapist dialogue was observed by one of the authors of this book. It illustrates the difficulties in achieving even the most limited kind of verification with a psychotic patient and the untoward results that strenuous ill-advised efforts in that direction can cause. The patient here was a 20-year-old university student who had been hospitalized for six days with paranoid schizophrenia, and the therapist was a first-year psychiatric resident.

Therapist: Douglas, we have talked about these voices that you hear continually. You feel they are real. Are you with me?
Patient: Yeah.
Therapist: Before we began to talk I clicked on this tape recorder. Every sound that is made in this room is being recorded on this tape. Right?
Patient: All right.
Therapist: We are going to demonstrate that these voices that condemn you and threaten you are only symptoms of your illness. If we can agree on that we'll have made a step forward. O.K.?
The patient remained silent.
Therapist: My voice has been recorded on the tape and so has yours. If the other voices really exist they too are being recorded on the tape. They'll come through loud and clear.
The patient moved uneasily and said nothing.
Therapist: We'll just sit here for ten minutes, with both of us saying nothing. If the voices are real they'll be on the tape.
Ten minutes passed.
Therapist: O.K. Now I'm going to rerun the tape from the beginning. You'll hear my voice and your voice. We'll see about those other voices.
The tape ran through completely.
Therapist: Well?
The patient rose, approached the still seated therapist and hit him hard in the face, almost knocking him from his chair. He turned and left the room.
No verification occurred.

This episode in an exaggerated way is a paradigm of the problems and limitations encountered in psychotherapeutic work with psychotic patients.

In recent decades the development of the various kinds of antipsychotic medications for schizophrenic, severely depressed, and manic patients has improved their prognoses greatly, and new concepts of therapeutic hospital environments have emerged during the same period. Most of these patients now recover, especially if treatment begins soon after the onsets of their illnesses. Psychotherapy is useful in aiding these patients to adjust well once more in the various activities that their illnesses interrupted, and it can help them find healthier ways of living in many areas of their lives. However, the schizophrenic patient must remain for years on a reduced dosage of his medication to avoid relapses. Most, but not all, depressed and manic patients can discontinue their medications once they return to their previous levels of feeling, thinking, and relating to others. Whether or not psychotherapy reduces the incidences of psychotic episodes in later years in recovered depressive and manic patients is an undecided question; the evidence is inconclusive at this time. Chapter 11 is entirely devoted to the subject of combining medications and psychotherapy; it is especially oriented toward the needs of nonphysician psychotherapists.

6 Energy Flows in Human Relationships

Human emotional and intellectual functioning often is conceived of in terms of mechanical models. For example, in Jungian psychology emotional activity is seen as occurring in the mind, which is viewed as being composed of concentric circles linked by arrows; the various circles are portrayed as housing the conscious mind, the ego, the personal unconscious, and the collective, or racial, unconscious. Freudian theory presents the mind, with its emotional and ideational activities, as a circle or irregular oblong that is divided by horizontal lines into conscious, preconscious, and unconscious areas, sometimes with arrows indicating their interactions. In later versions developed by Freud this circle or oblong is divided into the id, the ego, and the superego, and the space outside the circle represents a person's human and material environment. During the course of the twentieth century other conceptions of the structure of the mind, based on similar thinking but differing much in their details, have been proposed. Problem-oriented psychiatry's rejection of all such ways of looking at human feelings, thoughts, and interpersonal relationships was stated in Chapter 2, and the reasons for doing so were explained.

We feel that a viewpoint based on *energy flows* more realistically represents what goes on in people and in their relationships with one another. An example of this follows.

A hungry infant is lying on a wet diaper in a crib. Energy signals travel from its gastrointestinal tract, skin receptors, and other body tissues to his brain where many complex energy transformations occur. These cause impulses to reach the infant's vocal apparatus and other body regions, and it cries and thrashes. By sound and sight the flow of energy continues and reaches the mother. She, expending energy, comes to the crib, changes the diaper, and talks soothingly as she nurses the child. An interpersonal event has occurred.

Energy flows are much more complex in adults for they have acquired speech, mobility, large reserves of ideas and experiences, and skillful ways for interacting with people. If a man and a woman meet at a party, talk together, encounter each other many more times in various settings, and in time become lovers and have sexual intercourse, the number and variety of physiological, emotional, ideational, and interpersonal energy flows are immense. A single thought, such as "I like him," involves millions of bioelectrical exchanges in the brain.

By discussing these things in terms of observable energy flows, which can be studied and often measured, we are on sound scientific ground. Nothing abstract, speculative, or unprovable is involved, and any trained observer with the necessary equipment at hand can repeat these observations.

We can consider each energy flow in terms of its *source*, *course*, and *conclusion*. In the case of the infant the source of the energy flow lies in the physiological processes that create the child's discomfort, and the course runs through its fretting and crying to a conclusion in the mother–child activities at the crib side. In the case of the man and woman the energy source is the physiological readiness of each of them to be attracted to the other; the course travels through the details of their subsequent meetings, and the conclusion occurs in the intense sexual experience they have with each other. For purposes of illustration a great deal in each case has been simplified and abridged.

A person's usual kind of energy flow in a certain situation forms one of his personality features. Thus the things an infant does when it is in distress are characteristic of it and the things that happen at such times have significance for the future. What we have described above is a healthy energy flow and it ends in an interpersonal event. In other cases an infant's characteristic energy flow in such circumstances is different. If he is markedly autistic he lies wet, hungry, and cold in his crib with little fretting, or perhaps merely low moaning. He does not reach out for help and no interpersonal event occurs. It is this lack of outward energy flow that constitutes the most apparent aspect of a severe autistic disorder. Similarly, the energy flows in the man and woman sketched above characterize them. If one or both of them had been homosexual, his or her energy flow at the party would have been toward a person of the same sex and the conclusion would have been different.

The sum of a person's energy flows (combined with his well-being operations and other features) makes him the kind of individual he is and the kind of person whom others see. His healthy energy flows constitute his personality assets and his unhealthy energy flows, or the absence of them, form his emotional and interpersonal problems. Thus we can talk of obsessive-compulsive energy flows and phobic energy flows when energy flows find their conclusions in these kinds of clinical difficulties. Psychotherapy is to a large extent concerned with work on unhealthy energy flows.

An Example of an Energy Flow in Psychotherapy

In many cases the source of energy in an unhealthy energy flow lies in turmoil produced by interpersonal trauma in both past and ongoing relationships. For example, harsh, unaffectionate behavior by one or both parents throughout a child's formative years may leave much smoldering hostility in him. If abetted by later damaging relationships in his adolescence and adulthood, this may be a source of energy that produces a neurosis or a personality disorder. This is illustrated in the following patient–therapist dialogues; they trace the source and course of an energy flow to its conclusion in the patient's psychiatric difficulties.

The patient is a 38-year-old woman who is married and has a 16-year-old daughter. Her main symptom is an obsession that she will become psychotic ("go berserk and run wild") and will thereafter be permanently hospitalized. She has had this obsession for three months. Waves of severe anxiety, at times amounting almost to panic, sweep over her occasionally. She sleeps badly. Sleep, involving absence of vigilant self-observation, seems to her a possible precursor of the disaster that hourly preoccupies her. The patient is talking about her relationship with her mother as the dialogue begins.

Patient: My mother had to have everything just right all the time; everything had to be clean and in order. Each towel and washcloth in the bathroom had to be on its special hook or rack; if it wasn't she took it down, folded it neatly and put it in its place. All my clothes, even the ones I was wearing, had to be perfectly clean. She washed clothes until every spot was gone and then meticulously ironed them; if they didn't come out right she would start all over again. Sometimes the same blouse or pair of slacks would be washed, rinsed, and ironed three times. We could have afforded to have someone to do that kind of work, but she was never satisfied with anyone who came to work in the house; no maid or washerwoman ever lasted more than a few days.

Therapist: Did she say why all this was necessary?

Patient: She had certain sayings. "If a thing is worth doing, it's worth doing well." "A place for everything and everything in its place." "Cleanliness is next to godliness." And so on.

Therapist: How did you fit into all this?

Patient: A lot of the time she said all this work was my fault. She said I played carelessly and that my clothes were dirty half an hour after I put them on. Any grease spot from my bicycle, or a stubborn stain, would bring the house down on me. She said that if it wasn't for my carelessness she wouldn't have to be always drudging and that she was working herself into an early grave because of me. She would point to the few gray hairs on her head and say that I was the one who put them there. She said I kept her hands red and sore from all the washing with detergents and bleaches, and that my messiness, combined with indifference to her suffering, kept her working far into the night—washing the kitchen and the bathroom, vacuuming rugs, arranging clothes in drawers and closets, and ironing, ironing, ironing. She said that I would cause her to die before she was fifty.

Therapist: Did all this seem realistic to you?

Patient: I guess so. I heard it all my life. One of my earliest memories is of me sitting on a chair in the corner of the kitchen while she mopped the floor, talking endlessly. Somehow it was my fault; I had spilled jam or something on the floor. I couldn't have been more than three at the time. It was what I grew up with.

Therapist: Did she say the same sorts of things about your stepfather, or, earlier, about your true father?

Patient: I don't remember much about my true father. He and my mother were divorced when I was four. He moved to Louisiana and remarried. I've only seen him twice since then; my stepdad wasn't around much. During the day he worked and at night and on weekends he fiddled with his antique cars in the garage.

Therapist: What was your mother's health like during those years?

Patient: She complained constantly about her back and about headaches and stomach pains. She said they were caused by overwork. Sometimes she would go to a doctor but she never stayed long with any one of them. It was me, she said, that was the cause of it all, and what could a doctor do about that? She said that doctors just string you along, send you for lots of tests that always turn out normal, and that they are only interested in your money. A couple of them tried to send her to a psychiatrist, but she blew up at that and never went.

In tracing this turbulent relationship with her mother, and the guilt, worthlessness, and desolation she felt in it, we are exploring the interpersonal source of the energy flow that in time was to lead to her obsessive disorder.

Therapist: As the years went on did these things change in any way? Were there no variations in your relationship with your mother?

Patient: As I got into my teens it changed. She talked less about me and to me. She avoided me. She began to be silent and seclusive. At times she seemed afraid of me.

Therapist: Afraid?

Patient: Yes.

Therapist: Did she seem afraid of anyone else?

Patient: She seemed afraid of my stepdad too. She rarely left the house.

Therapist: Did your stepfather continue to be aloof and distant with you?

Patient: No. He took more interest in me as I grew up. He took me places. He did things with me.

Therapist: Such as?

Patient: He took me to baseball games and basketball tournaments, and when a big pop star like Elton John came to the Municipal Auditorium or the Starlight Theater he would take me to see him.

Therapist: Did your mother go?

Patient: No. He would invite her, but he didn't push it.

Therapist: Did she comment on his doing these things with you?

Patient: She said we got home too late. Only that.

Therapist: Too late?

Patient: Sometimes we went for a hamburger and a milk shake afterward, or for a snack at a night spot where they had live music, and didn't get home until one or two o'clock. She always waited up until we came in.

Therapist: Did she object to his increased interest in you?

Patient: No, not really.

The therapist remains silent, unwilling to probe, but feeling that the patient has more to say, if she can.

Patient: Well, she didn't like him kissing me.

Therapist: What did she say?

Patient: She said it was mushy.

Therapist: What did she mean by mushy?

Patient: He kissed me on the mouth . . . Hard.

Therapist: How did you feel about that?

Patient: I don't know. I was just a kid. Fourteen or so. He gave me presents, expensive things, clothes and fancy costume jewelry. When I was fifteen he began to do other things. He would walk into the bathroom when I was taking a shower or was on the toilet and say embarrassing things about . . . about my body. . . . He didn't act as a father should. He did things with me that . . .

Therapist: I take it that this is difficult to talk about.

Patient: Yes. There's more . . . awful things . . . that . . .

Therapist: (*Feeling that the patient is becoming too anxious to proceed on this subject, at least at this time*) This is a pretty tense topic. We won't go into it anymore just now. We'll simply say that this bothered you a great deal and that in some way it may have upset your mother. O.K.?

Patient: (*With a relieved smile*) O.K.

In this interchange the patient and the therapist have explored a source of the emotional turmoil, which in time led to her obsessive disorder. They also have moved imperceptively into tracing its course.

When the patient was 16 her mother developed a psychotic depression with bizarre paranoid features. Psychiatric hospitalizations and treatments resulted in partial improvements three times. Finally she was hospitalized in a state psychiatric hospital where she died of heart disease when she was 48. The patient was 20 at the time.

When her mother left her home to enter the state hospital the patient remained in the home for four months more. Then an aunt, her mother's sister, insisted that she come to live with her in a city several hundred miles away. The patient lived with her aunt until she completed her education and she married at the age of 22.

We move now to a later period of treatment as we follow the course of the energy flow that in time produced her obsessive illness.

Therapist: You appear to be a little listless today. We just seem to drift along.

Patient: I guess I'm tired. Earl and Mary Jo came in late last night and I watched TV until they got in. They went to see that English ballet company that's in town. Mary Jo is crazy about ballet. She has big pictures of ballerinas on the walls of her room, all in their bare feet. It seems they dance that way now.

Therapist: How long has Mary Jo been interested in ballet?

Patient: About a year or so.

Therapist: Is your husband also interested in ballet?

Patient: More or less. He likes to take her. He says it's part of his fatherly duties. "Be interested in what your teenager is interested in," the books say.

Therapist: Are you interested in ballet?

Patient: It's not my sort of thing, especially when you have to sit with your legs crammed up against the seat in front of you, if you're tall like I am. On video it would be all right, but these ballet buffs like to see it in the flesh.

Therapist: Was it hard to get Mary Jo out of bed for school this morning?

Patient: She was pooped, but she made it to school on time.

Therapist: How is Mary Jo coming along these days?

Patient: Fine. She's a pretty girl. Tall, mature for her age. She looks older than 16. She kids Earl, saying he's her boyfriend who takes her to expensive shows.

Therapist: How does Earl react to that?

Patient: He laughs. He jokes about her, says she has filled out in all the right places. He's proud of her. So am I.

Therapist: Does anyone else take her to the ballet?

Patient: The boys don't have that kind of money, and wouldn't spend it on ballet tickets if they did.

Therapist: Does Earl kid around with her in other ways?

Patient: Last week when she was going upstairs and he was at the foot of the stairs he pointed to her glued-on blue jeans and said she was pretty decorative to have around the house.

Therapist: How do you react to comments like this?

Patient: They make me uncomfortable, to use one of your words.

Therapist: Can you describe your discomfort a bit?

Patient: Sometimes I get the feeling that somehow I've been through this before. Not déjà vu, but something like that.

Therapist: Involving whom?

Patient: Barney.

Therapist: Your stepfather?

Patient: Yes.

Therapist: Can you talk further about this?

Patient: What happened between me and Barney couldn't happen between Earl and Mary Jo. Earl's an altogether different kind of man. And he's her true father, not her stepfather.

Therapist: In other words, history doesn't repeat itself.

Patient: Not in this case.

Therapist: This is sitting-on-the-edge-of-the-chair sort of stuff to talk about. However, I think it might be well to talk a little more about it.

Patient: It's like the dentist drilling, without Novocain.

Therapist: Do you think you can tough it out anyway?

Patient: Go ahead.

Therapist: Mary Jo is 16.

Patient: Yes.

Therapist: Is that an eerie, superstitious number for you?

Patient: I was 16 when mother got sick.

Therapist: And the way in which she got sick is the way you constantly fear you will get sick. Psychiatrically sick. With a bad ending. It sort of fits, doesn't it?

Patient: Yes. Anyway it's out now, between you and me.

Therapist: It might help to put this in context. This sort of problem is sufficiently common in psychiatry to have a name. The talion principle. An eye for an eye, a tooth for a tooth. What a person does to someone else will be done to him, or her, in the slow grinding of time. I mention this to indicate that what you suffer, and its causes, is not a weird, unique thing involving you alone. It's somewhat common. Getting it all out into the open, painful though it is, is a big step in getting well.

Patient: That's good news. I feel like I just had a tooth removed.
Therapist: Without Novocain.
Patient: Yes, but it's good to have it out all the same.

The course of this energy flow, and its conclusion in the patient's emotional disorder have been traced. There is much more work to do, but both the patient and the therapist can now see where they are going.

Other Aspects of Energy Flows in Problem-Oriented Psychotherapy

Energy flows often have their sources in childhood and the early years of adolescence; their courses, as well as their conclusions, as a rule occur in relationships and events of later periods. The conclusion of an unhealthy energy flow may be a personality disorder (as in undue passivity or anti-social behavior) or a neurotic difficulty (as in a phobia or an obsession) or, less frequently, from a statistical point of view, a psychosis.

The concept of energy flows conforms to twentieth-century ways of thinking about natural processes in general. As previously indicated in other contexts, Jungian, Freudian, and similar systems of thought are built on models drawn from Newtonian mechanics. They deal with spaces and their contents and with the interactions of one space on another. Twentieth-century thinking, beginning with Einstein and Planck, envisions everything in terms of energy and its movements. To think of emotional and interpersonal processes in terms of energy flows is therefore in keeping with current ways of thinking about both living and nonliving things. Energy flows also emphasize the continually changing nature of emotional and person-to-person life. Nothing is static. Nothing is ever jelled, even temporarily. This flexibility is yet another thing that makes psychotherapy possible by influencing the course and nature of ongoing processes.

Moreover, an energy flow gathers into one process and into one concept things that otherwise would be fragmented. It takes the place of libido, cathexes, mechanisms of defense, archetypes, various kinds of complexes, and many other things in other systems. An energy flow is a seamless progression that proceeds from its origin, or source, through its course to a conclusion. An energy flow also points toward the long future which stretches out beyond treatment and considers what effects treatment may have on marriage, relationships with children, vocational activities, social relationships, and cultural life.

7 Distortions and Deviations

In cases of prolonged intensive psychotherapy the therapist usually must sooner or later deal with distortions the patient makes in his relationship with him. For example, when the patient's main difficulty is characterological, as in an aggressive personality disorder or a withdrawn personality difficulty, exploring and resolving such a distortion is a major goal of treatment; it also is a prime avenue of therapy. In addition, behind each neurosis there usually is a characterological problem. The obsessive patient is at times a passive person and an anxiety-ridden individual may have one of various kinds of personality warps. In each case the patient's behavior in his relationship with the therapist is a distortion of the interpersonal situation, because the therapist has done nothing to evoke or merit such a reaction. The distortion is produced by the way the patient interacts with the therapist. The unduly passive person is placating and solicitous and the aggressive person is hostile and manipulating in spite of the fact that the therapist has in each case done nothing to produce such behavior.

This is illustrated in the following dialogue between a therapist and a paranoid patient.

Patient: I don't see how you remember all we talk about. You rarely make notes. Sometimes you don't make any at all.

Therapist: At the end of each session I write a short paragraph in each patient's record outlining what I felt were the most important things we talked about.

Patient: A short paragraph can't cover much of what goes on in 50 minutes.

Therapist: Does this bother you in some way?

Patient: I just don't see how you do it. Are our sessions recorded? Do you have a tape recorder hidden somewhere here?

Therapist: No, they are not recorded. Besides other disadvantages, it would be impossibly time consuming to listen to such recordings or to have them typed up for later reading.

Patient: You could just flick the recorder on whenever you felt we were talking about something important.

Therapist: That would distract me from giving full attention to the patient.

Patient: You're sure about that?

Therapist: Yes. You seem uncomfortable about this subject. Do you have some uneasy speculations about it?

Patient: No. But still . . .

Therapist: (*After a pause*) Still?

Patient: My boss said something to me on Wednesday that didn't sound right. He could only have said what he did if he had some sort of special information about me, like what I've talked about here.

Therapist: What did he say?

Patient: You don't already know?

The main difficulty that brought the patient to treatment has come to a head here and it has done so because of a distortion in his relationship with the therapist. However, this distortion offers the therapist special therapeutic opportunities. Dealing with paranoid patients, incidentally, is one of the most difficult problems in psychotherapy.

Distortions as Revealers of Historical Processes

Every distortion has a history. As a rule it begins in close interpersonal relationships during childhood and extends through adolescence into subsequent life. It is carried into all, or almost all, of a person's interpersonal activities. Thus the passive person in most of his dealings with people is passive and the aggressive person has a chip on his shoulder in all his associations. The reasons for these distortions come out as the patient's life history is examined. A person with a passive personality disorder often was reared in a household in which one or both parents were domineering and gave love only at the price of submissiveness. Relationships during childhood which might have had an ameliorating influence were weak or nonexistent. To the passive person submissiveness is realistic; it's the only way he knows to secure love and to be accepted. Difficulties arise in later life when his submissiveness leads to exploitation or clamps him in painful relationships from which he cannot extricate himself.

The concept of a distortion should be distinguished from the Freudian concept of transference. In transference the patient is believed to shift onto the therapist feelings and behavior once directed toward an important person in his life, usually one of his parents; he is believed to solve in the patient–therapist relationship things that were not resolved in the earlier one. The patient, according to this point of view, intensely relives his prior relationship in the one he forms with the therapist. Problem-oriented psychotherapy rejects this point of view. It holds that a person merely carries into many, perhaps all, of his relationships the customary ways he has for interacting with others, and these ways were formed in the matrices of earlier close relationships. He can have a helpful emotional experience in his relationship with the therapist, but he has it by developing new ways of relating to a person, and to people in general, rather than by reliving an earlier relationship.

This is illustrated in the following dialogue. The patient is a 24-year-old secretary who works in an office building near the therapist's office and she comes during an early lunch hour. By leaving her job a couple of minutes early and rushing to the therapist's office she is able to keep this appointment.

Patient: I've been waiting out there in your reception room for 20 minutes, after skipping my lunch period and rushing over here.

Therapist: I'm sorry. I'm running behind and . . .

Patient: If you couldn't see me on time why didn't you have your receptionist call me to come later, or cancel?

Therapist: I'm sorry but it wouldn't have been . . .

Patient: I suppose you're going to charge me for a full session.

Therapist: We can talk about that another time. We have something more important to talk about right now.

Patient: Like what?

Therapist: This isn't the first time I've kept you waiting and have shortchanged you on time, though it has never been intentional. This however is the first time you have talked about it. On other similar occasions what did you feel I might do if you talked about this?

Patient: Well, you might have stopped treatment, or maybe spaced the appointments out and gradually have gotten rid of me.

Therapist: In other words, if you had been assertive I might have retaliated—I might have rejected you?

Patient: I guess so.

Therapist: Has this happened in your life? Can you think of some relationship, particularly an early one, in which this occurred?

From the point of view of problem-oriented psychotherapy the patient has not transferred anything onto the therapist and she is not reliving anything. She has simply carried her customary ways of interacting with people into the treatment situation. Prepared by three months of therapy, she is ready to develop new ways of relating to people in this special, helpful type of relationship.

The Views of Problem-Oriented Psychotherapy on Erotic Developments during Therapy

In Chapter 4 we touched briefly on one aspect of this subject; we shall here discuss it more extensively.

Erotic developments during psychotherapy are distortions since the patient–therapist relationship is one of professional help and not a social one with sexual connotations. Erotic developments may be due to (a) characterological problems of patients who tend to eroticize many kinds of relationships or (b) special conditions that prevail in the treatment situation.

Erotic Developments as Characterological Expressions

Some persons tend to eroticize prolonged, close relationships in social, vocational, educational, and other situations. Eroticizing a relationship in some ways simplifies it; the person who transforms his vocational, social, or school situation into a sexual one no longer has to deal with the other person as a boss, coworker, or teacher in a mature and often taxing manner. He becomes a would-be lover, and vocational or academic work in the ordinary sense slows down or stops altogether. It is replaced by sensual attachment, admiration, and uncritical acceptance.

How does a therapist handle such a development when it occurs in psychotherapy?

Patient: I feel something special and important has happened between us during the time I've been seeing you. I think you've noticed it. You've become important to me as a person, as a man. There's no other way to say it. I'm in love with you.

Therapist: Have you considered what such a development might do to our treatment?

Patient: What do you mean?

Therapist: If our relationship as therapist and patient were to be transformed into a man-and-woman one any work on the difficulties which brought you to see me would slow down and perhaps halt altogether. I would cease to be of any use to you. I would stop functioning in the way in which you need me to function.

Patient: I don't see why.

Therapist: We couldn't talk about us in an affectionate way and also go on exploring your life and how it has produced your emotional problems. One of the two would have to go by the board and, if the erotic element dominated, it would be the treatment.

Patient: I don't see why we couldn't go on as before—some of the time.

Therapist: A problem like this occurs once in a while during treatment.

Patient: Problem? Do you think what I feel for you is only a problem?

Therapist: Perhaps we ought to consider the special circumstances of psychotherapy which sometimes lead a patient to feel the way you do.

From this point onward the therapist leads the interview into the channels discussed in the following paragraphs.

Erotic Developments Arising out of Some Special Circumstances of the Treatment Situation

The things we shall examine here apply to all therapists—psychiatrists, clinical psychologists, psychiatric social workers, and psychiatric nurses with special psychotherapeutic training.

We shall begin by asking a rarely voiced question. How often does a person over a long period of time spend from one to several hours each week talking without reservation about his or her life to another person whose defined interest is to be helpful? In no other relationship does a person have the same intensity of attention from another individual that a patient has and the same boundlessness as to what can be talked about. The therapist moreover is a well-educated, respected, economically comfortable person and he or she usually is addressed by the title "Doctor." In addition, in our culture a person tends to idealize any type of therapist he has, whether the therapist is a family physician, a medical specialist, or a psychotherapist. To think otherwise would be painful, for to think of one's therapist as careless, incompetent, or mercenary, when one's welfare is in his hands, would be devastating. As an elderly internist long ago expressed it to us, "The patients will idealize you if you give them half a chance." The average patient hence thinks of his therapist as a good, wise, skillful helper in whom he can place great trust. This strong cultural factor buttresses the other factors we have outlined here.

The following abridged dialogue illustrates one approach to this problem. The patient has just made an erotic declaration to the therapist.

Therapist: Have you considered the special circumstances of psychotherapy that sometimes are conducive to such feelings?

Patient: What do you mean?

Therapist: Twice a week you spend almost an hour talking with me about your feelings, thoughts, and experiences, and this has been going on for five months. Have you ever at any time in your life spent so much time talking about yourself without restrictions or limitations to another person?

Patient: I guess not. When you talk with other people they usually start talking about themselves and there are a lot of things they don't want to hear about.

Therapist: Has anyone in your life ever accepted you and what you say in such a noncritical way—without censure or judgment, but with only a willingness to help?

Patient: If other people did that I suppose there wouldn't be a profession like yours.

Therapist: Would it surprise you to learn that such feelings, call them erotic if you will, by a patient toward a therapist occur once in a while in our kind of work?

(*The therapist silently waits for the patient to continue*)

Patient: How long does this go on? It's real to me, and it hurts.

Therapist: One of my teachers said that in over forty years of psychotherapeutic work, and in other psychiatric practice, he had never seen such feelings persist if they did not become the major focus of therapy. He found that they usually become much less intense long before the end of therapy. In most cases they subside into a warm admiration of the therapist, and no more than that. It's like a Coca-Cola that you uncap and leave for a few hours in the refrigerator; it still has an agreeable taste but the fizz has gone out of it.

Patient: (*Laughing slightly*) You and your damned similes!

There are many things a therapist does not do to avoid precipitating erotic developments. He or she should avoid physical contact with a patient, such as helping him on with his coat or jacket at the end of a session. He should not give him rides home if he is the last patient of the day or lunch with him if he is the last patient of the morning; he does not comment on attractive clothing or a new hair style unless there is some special therapeutic reason for doing so, and he avoids staring at tight blouses and skintight blue jeans. In brief, he avoids all things that might be interpreted as suggesting a special nontherapeutic interest in the patient. There are exceptions, however. Some older, and especially European trained, therapists shake hands with all patients at the beginning of each session, and at times an infirm patient may be helped to his chair. Some therapists find it helpful to take adolescent patients to lunch, or to lunch with them in the office, and may in a friendly way drape an arm over an adolescent's shoulder at times. Work with children often involves disregard of many of these rules.

Administrative Manipulation of the Therapist as a Deviation in Therapy

Some patients come to therapists for mainly administrative reasons. The patient who comes after his boss has said, "You get help for your drinking if you want to continue working here," may be more motivated by financial factors than by a true interest in treatment. The sexual exhibitionist who is told by a judge, "You either see a psychiatrist and get straightened out or go to jail," may feel resentment about being in psychiatric treatment and therapy becomes a foot-dragging process. The drug user or kleptomaniac who is given the "treatment or jail" option by a law enforcement officer, the pedophiliac who is told by irate parents to enter treatment or face social exposure, and other persons who are sent after trouble on the job, at school, or in some other setting often see psychotherapy chiefly as an administrative procedure.

These are unpromising candidates for therapy. The only chance for true help lies in going into the administrative problem at the outset of treatment.

Therapist: How do you feel about treatment with me?

Patient: I didn't have much choice, did I?

Therapist: How do you feel about this lack of choice?

Patient: I don't like being railroaded into things.

Therapist: Would it be fair to say that you're angry about seeing me?

Patient: I guess so.

Therapist: If this anger persists it will be quite a problem in treatment. We'll find treatment a sluggish, tooth-pulling process. It may make treatment impossible.

Patient: What do you mean, impossible?

Therapist: Instead of discussing many things that have happened in your life and how they have led to this problem, we may end up in a sort of fencing match. Therapy can occur only if the patient has at least a certain amount of interest in it. He must do most of the work, which is talking about his feelings, thoughts, and experiences.

Patient: You'll get paid and it will only be for six months. After that the judge will forget about all this.

Therapist: I'm afraid that won't be good enough.

Patient: A young doctor like you can't be overloaded with patients. If you don't treat me somebody else will.

Therapist: I'm sure the court will be able to recommend someone else. I'd like to help you but it doesn't seem to be in the
cards.

A long pause ensues.

Patient: I'd rather stick with you. At least you're frank.

Therapist: Well, we'll give it a try. Can you tell me how you feel
in the hours or days before you go to the park to expose
yourself? For example, is there a slow build-up of tension,
or how is it?

In working with this kind of patient the therapist as a rule
must meet him more than halfway and be unusually active.
Rules given in the early chapters of this book often are broken
in the process.

A variant of such administrative deviations in therapy occurs when a patient comes to be treated until the time when
the therapist can give him a letter stating that he is free
("cured" in some cases) of the difficulty that caused him forci-
bly to be sent for treatment. There may be a specific time
limit; at times a letter must be forthcoming before the beginning of the next college year, or before the end of a stated
probationary period, or before some other event takes place.
In such cases the therapist should make it clear, as gently as
possible, that he or she cannot guarantee such a letter, especially by a set date, and that what the therapist can say in a
letter must be determined by treatment results and progress.

Factors in the Therapist's Behavior that May Influence Distortions in Therapy

Earlier in this chapter we briefly indicated a few things a
therapist should avoid doing in order to reduce the chances of
an erotic distortion in a patient. We shall now consider the
broader subject of how a therapist's behavior may cause a

variety of reactions in a patient, creating factitious feelings and thoughts in him. Such feelings and thoughts are factitious in the sense that the stimulus for them does not come from the patient's feelings and life experiences but are in response to the therapist's ongoing feelings, thoughts, and actions.

A simple example makes this clear. While taking her morning shower a therapist notices a large, fixed lump in her breast; when she gets to her office she calls her physician and makes an appointment for late that afternoon. Throughout the day the therapist is anxious, somewhat depressed, and less attentive to what her patients say and do; she often thinks about what her physician will say and what subsequent tests may reveal. As a result of her altered behavior one of her patients that day feels that she is becoming discouraged with him and is thinking of terminating treatment or of spacing out his appointments. Another patient feels that the therapist is becoming apprehensive that her depression may be deepening and that suicidal urges may be in the offing. Yet another patient, seeing the therapist for the first time about her upset adolescent son, may feel that the therapist's manner indicates that her son's problems are so marked that psychotherapeutic help has little to offer.

The manner in which each patient reacts during this day is largely dependent on the patient's personality and emotional difficulties, but the stimulus for his reaction is a disturbance in the therapist. This simple example makes plain that what goes on in psychotherapy is more complex than has been indicated up to this point in this book. We must now examine this new dimension.

A therapist should be constantly observing the interpersonal field in which he is working. For didactic purposes this field may be considered in terms of (a) the emotional and intellectual state of the patient, (b) the emotional and intellectual state of the therapist, and (c) the total therapeutic relationship, whose aim at all times is to help the patient.

Temporary Problems of the Therapist that May Cause Distorted Reactions in Patients

Some of the things that may upset a therapist and skew the interpersonal field are transitory. Many kinds of minor physical distress fall in this category. A therapist who is coming down with a bad cold or has a sore knee from a minor car accident while coming to work may be sufficiently different in his behavior that day to disturb his patients. What should a therapist do when he has such a discomfort? We feel he should briefly make this clear to the patient. "I'm coming down with the flu and if I seem different today it's not because of anything you have said or done. It's me." "I have a sore knee from a minor car accident while coming to work this morning. So if at times I frown or tighten my lips when I move in my chair it is not a reaction to what you are talking about." Most patients accept this well. It solves the problem.

The problem is more difficult when the temporary upset is caused by a person-to-person stress in the therapist's life. Let us assume that the therapist described above as finding a lump in her breast instead has an interpersonal disturbance that morning. While waking her 14-year-old daughter to go to school she notices that a small plastic sack full of white powder falls from under the pillow onto the floor. She feels that there is not enough time to go into the matter adequately with her daughter at that time and decides to delay discussion of it until the late afternoon. Or let us assume that while going through a drawer to find a belt to match her slacks she finds a crumpled bill for women's clothing that her husband bought at a fashionable shop and that never arrived in her hands or in her daughter's. In either case there may be a simple explanation. The white powder may be an alternative herbal medication a school friend gave her daughter to take for acne, and the clothing may have been her husband's birthday present for his sister in a distant city. But until the therapist finds this out that evening she will be tense and preoccupied as she meets her patients, and that may affect them adversely.

What does a therapist do in such a situation? We feel the answer is the same as for physical upsets, but the therapist does not reveal details of his or her private life. "If I don't seem to be on your wavelength quite as well today as during other sessions it is not because of anything you say or do. I had a small unpleasant surprise earlier today and haven't quite gotten over it. Now that that's out of the way, let's get down to work. Last time you were . . ."

Occasionally the disturbing element is a mechanical one. The air conditioning breaks down in the middle of a hot summer day or the heating system stops working when the temperature outside is below zero. Pneumatic drills on nearby building sites, the racket of defective power mowers on the grounds outside, and the shouting arguments of truck drivers over spaces in the parking lot below fall in this category. A brief recognition of the problem, perhaps coupled with a witticism, covers this relatively simple problem. "If I'm not on the ball as well as most times it's because of the freezing condition of this office. Keep your sweater and jacket on, as I have. Let's hope we don't have to put up umbrellas because of water cascading down from a broken pipe in the ceiling. O.K. Now perhaps you . . ."

Long-Lasting Problems of the Therapist that May Cause Untoward Reactions in Patients

When distortions in a patient's feelings and thoughts during treatment are caused by features of the therapist's personality the problem is much more complex. We feel it is better to address this subject in terms of specific true cases rather than in broad general statements. General statements tend to degenerate into platitudes. We knew personally the three therapists described below and at times examined persons who had been treated by them. These thumbnail sketches are selected from a spectrum that includes many kinds of difficulties. Most therapists are stable and effective, but therapists whose personality problems skew patients' reactions are sufficiently common to merit our attention.

Dr. Green, a psychotherapist in his late thirties, treated patients for various kinds of personality disorders and neurotic syndromes. He worked well with men but in his treatment of women he at times lapsed into abrasiveness and depreciation of them. Clinicians in the community who saw his former patients heard that he occasionally was impatient or annoyed with them. Women with marital problems often came away with the impression that they were the major contributors to their marital difficulties and that any problems of their children were due to the unhealthy home atmospheres they themselves had produced. He had two suicides of women patients within an eight-month period. In his personal life he was in his third marriage, his first two having ended in bitter divorces. Two of his colleagues jointly assumed the responsibility of talking to him about these things and they suggested that until he solved the problems he had in his attitudes and feelings toward women, he should restrict his practice to men. The only result was lasting coldness between Dr. Green and the two colleagues. Dr. Green cited the two years of psychotherapy he had had early in his career for both therapeutic and learning purposes.

A brief note should be inserted here on the limitations of boards that certify psychotherapists. A specialty board, by oral and written examinations and by observation of the candidate as he interviews a few patients, can judge his erudition and technical skill. It cannot, however, in so brief a time and by such limited contacts, evaluate his personality structure and any subtle problems in it that may affect his therapy. As a result there is a certain fallacy in such boards certifying to the public persons whom they cannot evaluate regarding such a crucial factor. A board can more validly certify a dermatologist, a surgeon, or a psychologist who does only psychological testing because in these cases the candidate's personality affects his practice to a much lesser extent. Two of the three psychotherapists we are presenting here had been certified by specialty boards.

Dr. Brown was a well-established psychotherapist in her late forties. Her self-confidence and her sense of her own importance had only vague limits. "Everyone knows that when I was at the Westmoreland Hospital and Institute I made the outpatient department the nationally known facility it has been ever since." "That paper I gave at the Philadelphia meeting two years ago is having a marked effect on what is done in psychotherapy in this country." Her capacity to spout or write platitudes, and to document them in the long lists of references at the ends of the articles she wrote, was impressive. Her self-assurance and dogmatism made her insensitive to some of her patients' needs and she rammed their feelings, thoughts, and experiences into whatever theoretical pigeonholes she was interested in at the time. Many of her patients were material for her next paper regardless of whether their problems were relevant to it.

She left a significant number of patients puzzled and anxious about what had gone on in their therapy, which she blandly assumed always to have been successful, and many of them sought later help in other hands. She had a dedicated husband and four adoring pubescent and adolescent children. Her older colleagues considered her either a wry joke or a hopeless caricature, but some of her younger colleagues admired her. No one, so far as we know, ever tried to talk to her about the unfortunate effects she had on an appreciable number of her patients; her self-assurance was considered to be impenetrable. When she died in an automobile accident in her middle fifties the obituaries in both professional and lay publications were long and fulsome. "In the untimely death of Dr. Elizabeth Romney Brown our profession has lost one of its outstanding . . . etc . . . etc . . ."

The third example, Dr. White, was the son of poor immigrants and he got his education only through extensive sacrifices by his parents and siblings. He married an ambitious woman and over a 20-year period they elbowed their way into the social elite of their city. Dr. White was a competent, dedicated therapist with well-to-do, socially prominent patients, but he was less helpful to lower-middle-class and working-class patients. They frequently had their appointments shifted to another time at the last minute to give elite patients more time, or hours that were more convenient for them, or to create space for a new such patient. Because of frequent occurrences of this kind (and many appointments were cancelled altogether for that week) patients from ordinary backgrounds often discontinued therapy with a vague sense (which they rarely could put into words) that something was missing in their treatment. Dr. White did not so much damage these patients as he failed them. The extensive personal psychotherapy he had had for both therapeutic and learning purposes did not solve a problem that treatment rarely identifies, let alone deals with. Is snobbism a personality problem or a socioeconomic one, or an intricate combination of the two?

We do not have pat answers to the many questions raised by these three psychotherapists and the many variations of them. Indeed, their existence indicates that no satisfactory solution to this general problem has yet been found. Only a small minority of psychotherapists have such personality difficulties; the vast majority are reasonably well adjusted by virtue of their original character structures and any therapeutic experiences they have had during their training or in the early years of their careers. In a book of this kind we can only indicate the existence of this problem. To consider it in detail and to speculate on solutions for it would require several chapters or perhaps form the material of a volume dedicated solely to it.

The Material Surroundings of Psychotherapy

We shall close this chapter by briefly considering how the material surroundings of psychotherapy may influence the feelings, thoughts, and reactions of patients toward a therapist.

A therapist should not have in his office things that reveal his personal life because such things may affect a patient's reactions. Each therapist must exercise a good deal of judgment on such details, but a good rule is when in doubt, don't. We feel it is best for a therapist not to have on his desk or wall pictures of his marital partner and children. Formal photographs tell a certain amount and informal or group photographs reveal much more. For example, erotic developments in therapy can be influenced by whether or not the patient knows the therapist is married, and the duration of that marriage is to some extent indicated by the apparent ages of children in photographs. Patients occasionally ask questions when such pictures are present. "Is that your wife (or husband)?" "How old are your children?" "I suppose you've only been married once?" No matter how tactful the therapist is as he or she declines to answer such questions ("We're here to talk about you, not me") it is still a dismissal and smacks of rebuff. It is also a limitation on what can be talked about, especially when the therapist has previously indicated that in therapy any topic can be discussed.

Sporting trophies, even when used as paperweights or book ends, provide easy digressions for patients when tense subjects are approached. "I suppose you're a golfer. What's your handicap?" Once more the therapist must either answer the question, wasting the patient's time and risking more golfing talk, or decline to answer it and run the risk of seeming to rebuff him. "I'm a bowler myself, Doctor. Do you bowl in a league?" It is hard to refuse to answer such a question without seeming, at least gently, to rap the patient on his knuckles. Trophies and similar decorations also suggest that the therapist is in good physical shape, or is trying to be, and may lead a patient to think of him or her as a lithe, muscular, agile person rather than as a therapist.

Lithographs, water color paintings, and photographs from the campus of his alma mater sometimes can trip a therapist up. "Is that Harkness Tower? My brother went to Yale and I visited him there a few times." "I notice that your college campus scene has palm trees on it. Did you go to school in southern California or Florida?" "That football team photograph on those college steps must have been taken when you were at college. You have the physique for that sort of thing." At the risk of seeming picayune we shall state that it is best not to wear a wedding ring for the same reason that pictures of marital partners and children should not be present. The absence of a wedding ring gives no information since many married people do not wear them, but the presence of one identifies the therapist as a married person, and one who, depending on the customs of his community, may be at pains to make it clear.

The therapist's office should be comfortable, but it should not contain things that smack of luxury. It should not have an oriental rug on the floor, sketches or paintings by identifiable, well-known artists, and framed autograph letters of historically prominent psychotherapists. They tell something about the therapist financially and perhaps reveal some of his tastes and interests. The best decorated office is one that the patient takes for granted and in which he doesn't notice anything in particular. These restrictions still leave a therapist wide fields from which to choose a few office decorations to avoid bare walls and Spartan austerity; a few decorations help an office to avoid a cold, institutional atmosphere and they give it a relaxed, comfortable tone.

In addition, an office in which nothing is expensive or out of the way allows the therapist to devote himself to his patient without intruding distractions. In a properly decorated office a therapist never reflects, "I hope she doesn't knock over that expensive lamp," or "Why does he have to track car grease onto a rug that cost me eleven thousand dollars?"

8 Special Techniques

In this chapter we shall discuss five special techniques in problem-oriented psychotherapy. They are (1) nonverbal communication, (2) management of deteriorating communication, (3) dreams, (4) the use of humor in psychotherapy, and (5) the patient's future as an area for exploration.

Nonverbal Communication

Nonverbal communication, whose importance we have noted previously in this book, is a two-way process. By it the therapist transmits information and attitudes to the patient and he should as much as possible be aware of the kinds of information he is conveying. The patient also is continually giving information though as a rule he does not perceive the information and feelings he is imparting. The most important things that occur in an interview are often nonverbal.

Patient: I think we should talk some more about the strong feelings I've developed toward you as a man, not just as a therapist.

Therapist: (Sits back in his chair, crosses one leg over the opposite knee and grasps his left forearm with his right hand in a lesser version of crossing his arms over his chest) We can talk about all your feelings here; that is part of the work we do.

In this interchange the therapist verbally said that this area is open for examination and at the same time said nonverbally that this is an unacceptable subject for discussion. Was the therapist aware that what he spoke was contradicted by what he did?

In the following dialogue it is the patient who cancels out nonverbally what he says in words.

Therapist: Do you find this a somewhat painful topic to talk about?

Patient: (Presses the flexed fingers of each hand down on the arms of the upholstered chair in which he is sitting, digging his nails into the surface; he briefly compresses his lips before answering) No, talking about this doesn't bother me.

Has the therapist gotten the nonverbal message the patient sent or has he accepted the patient's words at face value? If he gets the nonverbal information, does he feel that this area is too upsetting for the patient to explore for the time being or does he feel that it should be cautiously considered even if this distresses the patient? The important thing is that the therapist knows what is going on.

In other circumstances nonverbal communication permits a therapist to make a comment and allow the patient to accept it or not, depending on whether he is ready to do so. In a sense the patient can "pick it up" or not, depending on his psychological readiness.

Patient: I've always admired my father. The old man has guts and sticks to his guns until he gets what he wants. That's the main reason he's gotten to where he is. I'd like to be like that.

Therapist: (Tilts his head back and to one side, turns down the corners of his mouth, compresses his lips and elevates his eyebrows a little)

To most people these head and facial changes would say, "I doubt that and I wonder if you really mean it. Your father is an insensitive, domineering man who runs roughshod over everybody, including you." If the therapist were to put his wordless message into language, as has here been done, and if the patient were not ready to accept it, an impasse in therapy might occur. "Doctor, I don't think you understand my father. Beneath his gruff exterior. . ."

Nonverbal communication also gives a therapist a means for sharing feelings such as horror or shock with a distraught patient when words are inadequate.

Patient: When I went down into the basement I saw him in the dim light . . . hanging by an old chain from a pipe on the ceiling . . . his feet were still fluttering . . . his tongue and his eyes . . . Oh Lord! . . . I screamed . . . Sally came running and somehow got him down . . . He died before the ambulance came. How could I know he'd react that way to my telling him I was leaving him?

Therapist: (Narrows his eyes. A pained expression spreads over his face, with his eyebrows contracted and the skin stretched tightly over his cheeks. He silently looks at the patient with his shoulders and upper body inclined slightly forward.)

This in our opinion is better than saying, "How awful!" or "I know how devastating this was," or to trot out "I know just how you must have felt!"

Material objects sometimes can be employed in nonverbal communication. If after the dialogue above the patient continued to cry for several minutes the therapist might express understanding and patience by taking a box of Kleenex from a drawer and placing it on a table at her side. This says all that needs to be said at such a time.

We shall now complete the discussion of a subject which was broached in Chapter 1 but not fully considered there. Nonverbal communication can occur when a therapist is out of a patient's sight, as when he is sitting at the head of the couch of a reclining patient. In otherwise soundless rooms patients can hear the rustle of clothing as limbs move and body postures change. They may also detect the small sounds produced by upholstered chairs when body pressures are altered and when clipboards or notation papers are picked up or laid down. Many other slight noises can be perceived. There are in addition the voice tones, emphases, and rhythms of the therapist's speech, as well as coughs, throat clearings, and small clicking or smacking sounds of the lips and tongue. Patients in intensive prolonged therapy tend to develop, usually without being aware of it, expertise in perceiving these and other things in an out-of-sight therapist. One of the authors of this book recalls a patient who was being treated in an out-of-sight position; he one day asked, "Doctor, do you have a cold today?" The therapist honestly replied that he did not. Later that day he began to come down with laryngitis. The patient had been a closer observer of the therapist than the therapist had been of himself.

By such myriad nonverbal communications a therapist over a period of time may influence the kinds of material a patient discusses. It is as if the therapist were saying, "What you are now talking about is important in your treatment," or "This is not relevant to your problems and of little importance." Hence if the therapist feels that unconscious archetypes are important, he can over long periods of time lead his patient to talk on topics that support this point of view. If he feels that early parent–child lustful and hostile feelings are crucial he may by nonverbal means lead his patient to dwell on episodes in his life that seem to substantiate the therapist's position. The therapist may be unaware that he is influencing the material the patient brings to their interviews. In our opinion nonverbal communication is much more important in the apparent substantiation of psychological theories than often is recognized.

Nonverbal communication should be systematically taught during the training of psychotherapists, both for receiving information and for transmitting it. Videos, as well as step-by-step coverage of it in case supervision, should be used in this kind of teaching.

Management of Deteriorating Communication

A common experience in doing psychotherapy is that at one or more points in it the law of diminishing returns seems to set in. The sessions deal with trivial incidents and unimportant relationships. At such a time a psychotherapist should ask himself or herself a number of questions: Have I said or done anything, or failed to say or do something, that has resulted in treatment becoming painful for the patient? As a result, have excessive anxiety or guilt feelings been aroused, making it difficult for the patient to talk? Has some other distressing thing occurred?

Therapist: In recent sessions we seem to be dealing with things that are on the periphery of your life, things that don't pack much of a punch. Has therapy in some way become difficult or uncomfortable?
Patient: No, I don't think so.

Therapist: I've thought back about our recent sessions and this seems to begin about the time we talked about your fiancé.

Patient: Didn't I tell you about that?

Therapist: About what?

Patient: Four weeks ago we broke up.

Therapist: Did it hurt?

Patient: Yes, a lot.

Therapist: If it's not too upsetting maybe we should talk about that. How did it happen?

Here the therapist failed to pick up clues that an important relationship in the patient's life had gone wrong. The patient, who felt crushed and puzzled about what was going on in her life and her treatment, became silent and evasive. Since the patient did not talk about this relationship the therapist assumed it was going well. Pinpointing this onset of deteriorating communication revitalized therapy.

The following dialogue presents another instance in which a therapist failed to perceive something significant, and as a result communication began to decay.

Therapist: We seem to be skimming the surface of your life during the last three weeks. We don't appear to be talking about things that matter.

Patient: Maybe so.

Therapist: Did I say, or fail to say, something that bothered you?

Patient: You said that Marilyn was a support to me as I dealt with problems in my work and elsewhere.

Therapist: Did I get it wrong?

Patient: Support is about the last word I'd use in talking about Marilyn.

Therapist: Maybe I did get it wrong. If you had to choose a few words to describe her and pinpoint her personality, what words would you use?

In these cases the onset of deteriorating communication was abrupt and related to something specific. In other cases it is gradual and subtle.

Therapist: Do you get the impression that therapy seems to be running out of steam?

Patient: Well, perhaps.

Therapist: How long do you feel this has been going on?

Patient: I can't say. Maybe it started around the time of the holidays.

Therapist: We've been talking mainly about stresses in your work situation during the last couple of years. Did anything special happen around Christmas time?

Patient: My mother and her new husband came from Cincinnati to stay with us over the holidays and they've been here ever since. He drinks too much and tries to paw everyone, including me and Paula. Also he's out of a job. My husband wants to throw them out but he feels sorry for my mother. My feelings are all mixed up about them. My problems on the job have taken a back seat; the trouble's at home now.

Therapist: Maybe that's why therapy has been spiritless lately. How long has your mother been married to her present husband?

Was the former opinion that therapy was going well justified? In some cases the thing that has changed is not the nature of therapeutic communication but rather the therapist's opinion about it. He or she begins to realize that what he or she thought was vibrant, meaningful therapy, was not that at all. It was shadow boxing or thrust-and-dodge fencing or some other kind of pseudocommunication. At such times a therapist should think over all aspects of the case and perhaps talk it over with a colleague who can act as an impromptu supervisor. Such a person comes to the material fresh and may see things the therapist has misinterpreted or overlooked.

Is deterioration due to changes in the therapist's attitude toward the patient?

Therapist: Do you get the impression that lately we've been dealing with things that are superficial in your life, things that are really not significant—therapeutic chitchat, so to speak?

Patient: I guess so.

Therapist: Do you have any ideas about why we seem to have detoured onto this slow road?

Patient: I get the feeling you're a little discouraged about my progress.

Therapist: Can you put your finger on anything I've said or done that gave you that impression?

Patient: No.

Therapist: Has anything changed in the way I act or talk?

Patient: Not really. . . . It's just that when an appointment gets canceled because of bad weather or sickness in one of my kids or an emergency in your schedule, you let that session go and leave our next one for the following week.

Therapist: And before that I used to manage to make another appointment for you in the same week?

Patient: Usually. I know that my fears are about as bad as they've always been, and I suppose you want to work with patients you can help more. I can understand that, but still it's a little discouraging.

The therapist has a job cut out for himself, and it should not have been the patient who pointed it out to him.

Are one or more persons in the patient's life attempting to discourage him from continuing treatment, or perhaps even advising him to terminate it? This is more common than is often realized and patients frequently do not bring it up unless the therapist asks.

Therapist: Is anyone in your life saying anything about treatment that causes you to have more difficulty recently in talking here?

Patient: My uncle says I'm all right now and wants to know why you keep having me come to see you.

Therapist: Does he say anything else?

Patient: He says that from now on you need me more than I need you.

Therapist: And what do you think?

Patient: My uncle doesn't know much about my problems. Still, he swings a lot of weight in our family.

Here is another case from our files:

Therapist: We seem to have a hard time keeping these sessions going now, and you seem hesitant at the end of each interview about making the following week's appointment.

Patient: I'm having a few problems in coming to see you, and they're going to get worse.

Therapist: Can you tell me about one or two of these problems?

Patient: There's only one big one, but it's so big that I've been trying to taper treatment off. My father is opposed to my coming anymore and says that this month is the last one he's going to pay for.

Therapist: Ouch! Let's talk about this and see if we can work something out, and in the process maybe we'll learn something about your relationship with your father.

There are other circumstances in which persons in patients' lives try to dissuade them from continuing therapy. The marital partner who has long dominated and manipulated a patient with a passive personality disorder may begin to talk against treatment as the patient makes progress and becomes more assertive. Parents who were in favor of an overly dependent adolescent or young adult child entering into treatment may try to deter him from continuing it when he starts to move out of the parental home for the first time in his life. The spouse of a patient who is abusing drugs or alcohol may try to subvert therapy when the patient is no longer a depreciated, ineffective person but is becoming an achieving one; the husband or wife may have unhealthy needs that are met by having an inadequate partner. These factors may in fact have contributed to the person marrying an individual who abused drugs or alcohol.

Is therapy failing to fulfill the patient's expectations? "I've learned a lot about myself and in some ways I like myself more, but I'm still using crack as much as ever and that's why I came for help." "I get along much better at home and I've gotten rid of that motorcycle that I was going to kill myself with. But I'm still flunking out of school and can't settle down and study, and that's what my folks want you to change, and so do I."

Is a slowing down of communication in treatment a sign that the patient has made substantial progress and that treatment should move toward termination? A therapist from time to time should take a bird's-eye view of a course of treatment and examine where he and the patient are. At such times, when deteriorating communication is occurring, such an evaluation may indicate that treatment goals have been largely met or soon will be, and moves toward termination should begin.

In occasional cases of this latter kind the therapist, who may be in any age group, should ask himself, "Are the empty hours in my schedule causing me to hang onto this patient too long?"

Dreams

Dream interpretation is not much employed in problem-oriented psychotherapy. We shall, in numbered order, explain why this is so.

1. There are marked differences of opinion among equally erudite and experienced psychotherapists about the meaning of the same dream material, and there is no scientifically valid way for resolving these differences of opinion. For example, after hearing or reading an account of the same dream, and hearing what the dreamer said as he uninhibitedly spoke about it for a time, a Freudian may say that it expresses some aspect of the Oedipus complex; a Jungian may say that it reveals an inherited archetype in the collective racial unconscious such as the wandering hero; an Adlerian suggests that it reflects some facet of an inferiority complex; a Rankian states that it discloses a feature of the birth trauma; and a follower of some more recent writer on dreams may give it still another meaning. What is an uncommitted psychotherapist to do, especially if he asks, "What is the scientific evidence, verifiable by sense-observations in repeatable experiments or situations, which proves that any one of these interpretations is correct?" He receives either no answer or a decidedly unsatisfactory one.

2. A dream is a nonsensory experience, and to be studied scientifically any kind of experiential phenomenon must be observable by sense-observations such as sight, hearing, touch, and so forth. A person does not see, hear, touch, or otherwise perceive a dream. It is a purely internal experience. It is this feature of dreams that forever removes the study of their content and meaning from the realm of scientific investigation. Observers can validly study aspects of dreams other than their content and meaning. For example, by electroencephalographic means the frequency of dreams during a night's sleep, the lengths of individual periods of dreaming, and various other things can be investigated but these tell us nothing about the content of a dream. Only the dreamer can report the content of a dream

and, as we shall see, there are difficult problems in evaluating what he reports.

3. There are marked problems in evaluating the reliability of accounts people give of their dreams, and these problems throw doubt over the content of any particular dream, or of dreams in general. In other words, did the person really experience in his dream what he reports, or is he inadvertly giving an inaccurate account of it? Consider this from the viewpoint of waking experiences. A major task of psychotherapy is to help a person perceive what has happened, and is happening, in his life. (Some psychotherapists would say that this statement constitutes a definition of psychotherapy, or at least a crucial aspect of it.) If people have so much difficulty observing what has gone on and is going on in their waking lives what are we to think of experiences that are made much less accessible by the fact that the observer is asleep?

   Moreover, dream experiences cannot be corroborated or verified by anyone except the dreamer. In contrast, in waking interpersonal and emotional life the accounts of others with whom a person interacts can, if necessary or desirable, be obtained. In summary, if people quite sincerely misreport, and in a sense misexperience, what occurs in their waking lives, shall we not expect that the same thing probably occurs in an exaggerated degree when they report their sleeping experiences?

4. A further difficulty is made clear in the following abridged clinical vignette. A patient tells a psychotherapist that he dreamed that a rabbit was being attacked by a fox. The therapist instructs the patient to say without hesitation or omissions all that comes to his mind as he thinks about both the items of the dream and the dream as a whole. The patient, a man, says that it makes him

think of large vicious animals attacking small helpless ones, of powerful people exploiting powerless ones, of a brutish man criticizing a cowering boy, and of his father cruelly censuring and depreciating him. The therapist then says (in this abridged illustration) that these last words reveal the meaning of the dream, and in this episode of dream analysis a group of feelings, thoughts, and experiences that formerly was unconscious has become conscious.

At this point a person who has observed this event says, "I do not agree. I think that these last words constitute a new thought that has occurred during the patient's ongoing experience in talking with you. I see no evidence that this thought existed, either in this form or in some modified unconscious form, previously. In addition, I don't think that it is connected with the dream except in an inconsequential way." How is the dream analyst to disprove this statement? On the other hand, how is the skeptical observer to prove his statement? The answer is that neither one of them can prove his statement or disprove the statement of his opponent. This situation exists because, as indicated above, a dream is a nonsensory, purely inner experience and as a result lies beyond the realm of scientific inquiry.

For these reasons problem-oriented psychotherapy is hesitant to accept evidence based on dream analysis and rarely employs it. It feels that the only sound bases for psychotherapy are the feelings, thoughts, and experiences of patients that occur in observable interpersonal relationships. If psychology, psychiatry, and psychotherapy are to evolve into truly scientific disciplines they must concentrate on such data and eschew material that is forever destined to lie in the realm of speculation and uncertainty.

If a patient feels a need to talk about one or more of his dreams the therapist accepts this; he permits him to talk briefly or at length about his dream since a dream is, after all, an experience. However, the therapist views the dream as a starting point for whatever discussion follows its reporting and feels that the things the patient says do not necessarily reveal any particular meaning of the dream itself. In the example cited above it is relevant, and probably important, in the patient's therapy that he discusses his conflicts with his father, but this does not mean that linking such difficulties to a dream is the only or indeed the best way of approaching this aspect of his life.

The Use of Humor in Psychotherapy

Some therapists can employ humor skillfully in their work. In our opinion the kind of humor that can be used most effectively in psychotherapy falls in one of three categories.

1. In some instances humor consists of taking a common weakness or problem and expressing it pithily. Mark Twain had a special skill in this. "Giving up smoking is the easiest thing in the world. I know. I've done it a thousand times."
2. In the second type the humorist in a few well-chosen words unmasks human pretentiousness or debunks the dignity of authoritative, impressive persons. The American humorist Will Rogers once made a bet that he could, upon being introduced to him, get a laugh from President Calvin Coolidge, a man known for his aloofness, taciturnity, and austerity. When presented to President Coolidge, Rogers bent forward, cupped

his ear, and said, "Pardon me, I didn't catch the name."
He won his bet.

3. The third type of humor comes from getting sudden relief from pent-up feelings, such as hostile or sexual ones, which would otherwise not achieve expression. Slapstick, in which people are tripped up or outrageously insulted, is an example of this.

Each of these three general types of humor is of course much modified in style when utilized in psychotherapy.

Other forms of humor tend to misfire in psychotherapy. This is particularly true of humor that depends on sarcasm, irony, or oblique attacks on people that border on cruelty. Patients in such cases may apply the humorous remark to themselves and may feel depreciated or humiliated.

Humor is especially useful in certain therapeutic situations. For example, when interviewing parents who are discouraged or depressed about the problems of their adolescent children a therapist sometimes can throw these difficulties into a broader perspective by citing the old wry psychiatric adage, "Adolescence is not a stage of life; it is a psychiatric diagnosis." This stresses the commonness of such trouble and on the whole its good prognosis. On similar occasions a therapist may again quote Mark Twain: "When I was eighteen I thought my father was the most ignorant man in the world; when I was nineteen I was astonished at how much he had learned in only one year." Another quotation from Mark Twain which from time to time is relevant to parent–child conflicts is, "Adam was only human—this explains it all. He did not want the apple for the apple's sake, he wanted it only because it was forbidden."

A therapist in working with teenagers can sometimes provoke a laugh by reflecting resentment against parents and authoritative figures by referring to them as "super-dad," "super-mom," and "super-boss." Some adolescent–

adult confrontations are humorous when you take a few steps back and look at them objectively. "What goes on in your house sounds as if half the time things from *The Dinosaur Family* or *The Simpsons* were going on."

A type of humor that we occasionally employ with patients who have severe anxiety attacks, bordering on panic, is illustrated in the following dialogue. In our hands it works.

Therapist: Mr. Madison, I think that at this point I should tell you what is wrong with you. I think you can stand it.
Patient: O.K.
Therapist: I hope I don't confuse you with a lot of complicated medical terminology. Mr. Madison, (*the therapist proceeds in a slow, emphatic manner with well-chosen pauses*) your diagnosis is . . . what you suffer from . . . is what we doctors call . . . *scared shitlessness.* That is your diagnosis and that is what is wrong with you. I hope you can understand those words.
Patient: (*Smiling or laughing*) Yes, doctor, I think I do.
Therapist: When these waves of marked anxiety come over you and you feel that panic may be just around the corner, remember that you are merely *scared shitless* and that you are suffering from that dire medical disorder that is called *scared shitlessness.* A lot of people find that useful in taking the edge off such episodes.
Patient: I can see how they do.
Therapist: Your wife is very worried about you. Tell her your diagnosis, and if she doesn't believe I said such a thing have her call me on the telephone to have it confirmed. When you have one of these spells it doesn't help to have her sitting there looking almost as scared as you are. Also tell her that you will not go off the deep end and go berserk in one of them. There is about as much chance of that as there is of it happening to me or my receptionist, and I think we're hanging on pretty well.

When patients can laugh at a problem that frightens them badly they have taken a big first step in solving it. A therapist who feels squeamish about the word shit should recall that Chaucer employs it in *The Canterbury Tales.* An elderly psychotherapist, the late Tom Ainsworth, once explained to us why otherwise refined ladies at times use this word: "They deal with so much of it while changing diapers."

In some instances one of a patient's difficulties consists of feelings of inferiority and inadequacy in the workplace, in social gatherings, and in other situations. In these cases the therapist sometimes can put otherwise awesome, imposing people into perspective, and in so doing cut them down to realistic size, by posing the question, "How would all those people look if they had no clothes on? Just think of all those potbellies, drooping breasts, sagging bottoms, and spindly legs. The mind boggles!" In a similar situation a therapist may cite the remark that a fellow worker of one of our patients made after being bawled out in front of others by a domineering supervisor: "Excuse me, Mr. Christ. I didn't recognize you without your beard." A patient probably will never say this to a boss (he might be fired if he did), but in future such incidents he may remember these words, smile inwardly, and pass the event off without feeling abashed or devastated. At other times a brutal boss, teacher, or parent can be stripped of his terror by giving him a nickname: "Well, Ms. Maxwell, what has King Kong been up to lately?" We recall one family in which a tyrannical, ranting father was robbed of much of his awesomeness by referring to him as Hitler.

When a patient is inhibited by exaggerated respect for a therapist, or even has a certain dread of him or her, the therapist sometimes can diminish such feelings by referring to himself as a "head shrinker," "a shrink," or "a member of the head shrinkers' union." Once in a while a patient doubts a therapist's reassurances; he may feel that the therapist is trying to give him self-confidence by hiding "the awful truth" from him. At such a juncture a therapist may cock his head to one side and say, "I only lie to patients on Tuesdays, and today is Friday." When a patient is unduly upset about some moral pecadillo the therapist may find it useful to recount Mark Twain's story about his first lie. It occurred, he said, when he was 4 days old; he screamed to convince his mother that a diaper pin was sticking him when in reality he merely wanted more attention.

Some therapists utilize humor effectively and some do not. In the hands of the latter it may be counterproductive, and the patient may feel that the therapist is a frivolous person who does not take his problems seriously. The difference between a therapist who can employ humor well and one who cannot probably lies in nonverbal accompaniments, voice tones, and timing. In our opinion these things cannot be taught; they must be unplanned and spontaneous. Timing is important; the humorous interpretation that strikes home at one point may go badly astray a minute or two later. Pauses also are important; a slight pause, often just before the "punch" word or phrase, is critical. All these things are products of the therapist's personality, outlook on life, and lifetime background.

The Patient's Future as an Area for Exploration

It is sometimes useful in psychotherapy to cast an eye forward into the patient's future. The object always is to gain new insights into his or her current life.

Therapist: If you were to look forward to what you will be doing and how you will be living ten years from now, what would you see?

Patient: Many things, I suppose, will be the same. Except my marriage.

Therapist: How will your marriage be different?

Patient: I'll be in another one. I long ago decided that. The kids will be pretty much grown up then, and I'll be free to make a change.

Therapist: Each time we've touched on your marriage you've indicated that it was all right, and that there were no big problems in it.

Patient: Well, in a sense that's so. And that's what's wrong with it. I've seen that since the kids were little.

Therapist: I don't think I follow you.

Patient: Nothing ever happens with Max. One day is just like another. Year in and year out, it's always the same.

Therapist: Dull? Flat?

Patient: Yes, and I want more than that.

Therapist: What more?

Patient: I want a marriage with a surprise in it once in a while. Max is so stable, so predictable, so . . . solid.

Therapist: How would you like Max to change?

Patient: Max isn't going to change. I've tried. I long ago gave up hope of that.

Therapist: Still, how would you like him, and your marriage, to change?

Patient: No more of those damned fishing vacations we go on, and those roses, always red ones, on my birthday, and the potted hyacinths and chrysanthemums at Easter, and a black sexy nightgown at Christmas, and I wish he'd call me something besides "honey" once in a while. Everyone tells me how lucky I am to have a husband like Max. If they only knew!

Therapist: Are you sure you'll be happier after a change?

Patient: If I'm not I can always go back to Max. He'll wait. That's what's wrong with him. I know his every next move.

Therapist: We've gotten rid of most of the uncomfortable things that brought you to see me. What would you think of

shifting gears and turning this into a kind of marriage counseling—with you and Max coming to see me jointly?
Patient: Nothing will come of it. He'll agree to everything and he'll do everything you suggest—for two weeks—and then it'll be back to what it was.
Therapist: You may be right, and you may be wrong. Let's try it.

In some instances, however, looking into the future is too threatening or too devastating, and it should not be done.

Therapist: How do you see your life ten years from now?
Patient: I guess Martha will be pretty bad.
Therapist: Pretty bad?
Patient: I've done a little reading about Parkinson's disease.
Therapist: And?
Patient: It's awful. As the years go by the medications work less and less, and the shaking is replaced by rigidity of the whole body. They just lie there, "prisoners in their own bodies," as one book said, unable to do anything for themselves or for anybody else, and it may go on for years and years. And they know what's happening all the time. My God! I don't think I'll be able to stand it. I know euthanasia is against the law, but . . .

There is, we feel, no therapeutic goal to be gained by examining a future like that. The patient may be helped by comprehensive counseling, but only when the time comes.

9 Some Further Aspects

In this chapter we shall examine six special aspects of problem-oriented psychotherapy. They are (1) the extent to which an interview or a course of treatment should be deliberately organized, (2) examination of the patient's view of himself, (3) the role of advice, (4) investigation of abrupt changes and gaps in the patient's life, (5) the threefold nature of each person-to-person relationship, and (6) some broader aspects of problem-oriented psychotherapy.

To What Extent Should an Interview or a Course of Treatment Be Deliberately Organized?

In all the preceding chapters we have dealt with the ingredients of an interview and of a course of treatment. We shall now draw these things together and consider the extent to which an interview and a course of treatment should be structured. By this we mean the extent to which a therapist should make a planned effort to organize what occurs.

Some therapists feel that almost no deliberate organization should occur, and that the patient should be allowed to talk in as uninhibited and spontaneous a way as possible. This point of view posits that any steps by a therapist to make a systematic survey of the patient's problems, emotional life, and interpersonal world introduces an artificial, distorting element. While recognizing some merit in this concept, we disagree. We feel that in the first interview or two a therapist should obtain at least a bird's-eye view of what brings the patient to see him, the kind of person he is, and the milieu in which he lives. We also feel that as therapy thereafter progresses the therapist should have at least general ideas about its goals and the possible ways of achieving them.

A completely permissive approach sometimes goes badly astray and may even have unfortunate consequences. We recall the workup and therapy of a family in a child guidance clinic in which no systematic inquiries occurred and only spontaneously verbalized material was obtained. After the child and both his parents had been seen in weekly sessions for eight months it was discovered that the most disturbing, and disturbed, member of the household had not so far been mentioned; until this point her existence had not been known. She was the mother's mother, grandmother of the child, and mother-in-law of his father; she lived in the home and kept all its members in turmoil. Everyone found her so painful a topic that no one spoke of her. Eight months of therapy had passed in shadow boxing. The same thing can occur in individual therapy.

In the first session we usually begin with a general question that is little more than an invitation to talk. "Perhaps you might begin in whatever way seems best and most comfortable to talk about your difficulties." After the patient has, in response, been talking from 20 to 25 minutes it is evident whether he can in a reasonably clear way outline his problems, talk about who he is, and sketch out the interpersonal environment in which he lives. If he cannot do this we feel that the therapist should intervene and by questions and comments get the data he needs for evaluation of the patient. To allow the patient to wander from topic to topic, and from one group of feelings to another, accomplishes little in terms of the needs of the first interview or two. To continue in this manner for several sessions, or for weeks or months, is often a waste of time and occasionally is dangerous. A patient so treated on occasion may attempt suicide or do something that is socially disastrous and that could have been avoided if the therapist had known more about him. A reasonably systematic survey usually prevents the occurrence of conferences in which relatives say, "Do you mean to say that you saw him every week for five months and didn't know that since Christmas he has attempted suicide twice?" Or "Didn't you know that three months ago she lost her job and was so upset about it that she decided to see you?"

If an initial interview is fairly advanced and we are not getting at least a minimally coherent concept of the patient we pick up a clipboard and say, "Perhaps I might ask a few questions to orient myself about you, your life, and your difficulties. As we talk I'll make a few notes. It's hard to remember what kind of work a patient does, the kind of situation in which he grew up, his marital status and so forth, without making a few notes." Most patients accept this well; they accept it as one of the realities of clinical work. This step-by-step note-taking may continue for only 20 minutes or so in many cases; in others it extends beyond the end of the first interview into the second one.

We inquire why the patient has come to see us. That is, we elicit his "chief complaint," or "presenting problem." This, if taken at face value, may be misleading but it nevertheless gives useful information. For example, an alcoholic may say,

"I'm nervous and my boss insisted that I see someone," or "My husband is the worrisome type; he worries about everything and coming to see you was mainly his idea."

We also get a brief outline of the patient's life. How old he or she is, how many people were in his childhood home and who they were, what the major personality characteristics (as he sees them) of these persons were, whether he is married and whether this is his only marriage, how long he has been in his present job and how he gets along with other people in it, how many jobs he has had in the last fifteen or twenty years, and whether he is in good physical health. In regard to the last item, it at times is important to know that he has had a serious heart attack, or that he daily takes medication for a tendency toward epileptic seizures or has had four major automobile accidents that required hospitalizations.

We also inquire whether the patient has ever seen anyone in the mental health field for evaluation or for psychotherapy or for any other kind of treatment. If there is a history of such contacts we indicate that it frequently helps to get a report from that source. We have at hand a permission form in which the patient's full name and age and the approximate date of the previous professional contact are filled in and the patient is invited to sign it. However, if the patient's face and manner indicate hesitation about our getting such information we explore the patient's feelings on the subject. Some patients want a "fresh evaluation" that is "unprejudiced" by what other mental health workers thought about him, and in these cases we drop the matter, at least for the time being. A good deal of time is then spent in getting a detailed history of the patient's major difficulty—how it began, how it has progressed, and what his or her present condition is.

As the first or second interview comes to an end (and in many cases we do this at the end of interviews throughout a course of treatment) we frequently give the patient a "formulation" or "summing up." "Today we've taken a look at what goes on in your job and we've seen that the same erratic aggressiveness that causes you trouble in other areas of your life causes you problems there." Or "As we get a more detailed view of your relationships with your children it seems that there are problems in them that we ought to explore. Until now we have talked mainly about your early life and how its experiences contributed to your marked tendency to body overconcern and ruminations about possible ill health. Perhaps it is now time to shift our attention to current interpersonal difficulties." Such summaries are useful to both the patient and the therapist; they point to what has been done and what is yet to be accomplished.

However, a therapist should never "take over" an interview and stifle the patient's spontaneity and verve. The patient should always be allowed to roam widely in talking about his feelings, thoughts, and experiences. The one restriction is undue repetitiveness. Going over the same thing a few times may be useful, but beyond that it rarely is so. We feel it is unwarranted to allow such repetitiveness to be justified as "ego support," "working through," "talking it out," and so forth. When this rule is violated the words "muddle" and "morass" come to mind.

In occasional cases a course of treatment should be clearly structured. "Ms. Oates, I think it will be useful for you to have a counselor during your divorce and the period immediately after it. It is upsetting you a lot and you are going to have many decisions to make about yourself and your children as you carve out new lives for all of you. Basically you are a healthy person, but this is a stressful time." Or "Mr. Rodrigues, you've had a good business career; you were a top salesman. But now you're retired. You feel adrift, lost, and defeated. You've always viewed yourself as someone who could size up a challenge and meet it easily, and you see people like me as 'crutches.' Retirement is the most difficult adjustment many people make during their adult lives and a counselor who has experience in working with people making this adjustment can be helpful. We know what our goal is—comfortable, satisfying living under altered circumstances—so let's get to work on it."

At the end of each interview our parting words usually are "Good-bye *for now.*" This indicates that the parting is only an interruption in an ongoing process and is better, we feel, than simply "Good-bye" or an equivalent phrase.

However, therapy usually progresses without rigidly structured goals. Its aims are defined, and often redefined, as the patient's life is explored. The one set thing is the general aim—to help the patient get better. Everything else is fluid and flexible once therapy is well under way.

Examination of the Patient's View of Himself

It is sometimes useful at some point in therapy to examine how the patient sees himself or herself and then test out that view against reality. It has three aspects—how the patient sees himself, how others seem to see him, and how he is seen from the vantage point of the insights gained in treatment.

The patient in the following condensed dialogue is 16 years old.

Therapist: Susan, sometimes it is useful to talk about how you view yourself. If you were to describe Susan Adams to someone what would you say?
Patient: Well, I'd say that I am reasonably good looking, at least most people think so, that I do well in school, that I get along well with people most of the time, that I want to be a career woman, and so on.
Therapist: Only a career woman?
Patient: Yeah.

Therapist: You don't consider combining a career with marriage?

Patient: I can do without that.

Therapist: Are there things about marriage that you don't like?

Patient: The gooey stuff.

Therapist: What kinds of gooey stuff?

Patient: All of it.

Therapist: Kissing?

Patient: It begins with that.

Therapist: What is gooey about kissing?

Patient: Well, to begin with, all the things the boys want to do with their tongues while the kissing is going on. And their hands get busy at the same time.

Therapist: Do your girl friends share your views about this?

Patient: No, they claim they like it.

Therapist: Claim?

Patient: Well, I guess they do.

Therapist: Do you have a small problem here?

Patient: I don't see that I do. If I want to be a career woman, what's wrong with that?

Therapist: Nothing is wrong with it, so long as you have a choice, a comfortable choice.

Patient: What do you mean?

Therapist: That you are equally comfortable with a career and with the gooey things the boys like. If either one of these two possibilities is blocked by discomfort, then you're locked into the other. Do you see what I mean?

Patient: I guess so.

Therapist: People in my kind of work are great believers in choices. Options is the going word for it just now. If we could work on this, and if you'd develop the capability to keep your options open you'd be the richer, the better, for it. At least that's how it looks from where I sit. What about it?

Patient: Go on. I guess that's what I'm here for.

In the next dialogue the therapist and the patient explore how other people view the patient. The patient is a 38-year-old salesman.

Therapist: Sometimes it is useful in treatment to examine how other people view the patient. How do people, in general, see you?

Patient: When I'm on the road I'm a hale fellow well met. I'm always joking and cutting up. I always grab the check at lunch and I hand out invitations right and left for more of the same whenever customers are in town.

Therapist: And?

Patient: And when they come to town I'm not like that. They want to know where's that wonderful guy they knew in Topeka or Wichita and they can't find him, even when he's right in front of them. I'm a sort of Jekyll and Hyde, I guess.

Therapist: Is this a problem?

Patient: Yeah, 'cause the glum side of me is what's on whenever I'm not selling somebody building materials. My wife complains about it. "Why is it other people tell me you're the life of the party and all I ever see is you crumpled up in front of the TV?" And the kids are beginning to say more or less the same thing.

Therapist: Would it be better to try to get these two sides of you evened out a bit?

Patient: You've got your work cut out for you if you want to try to do that. I've always been like this.

Therapist: *We*'ve got our work cut out. If we only get the job half done it will still enrich the lives of your wife and kids, not to mention the customers and *you*.

In the next interchange the patient examines herself from the viewpoint of the insights she has developed in therapy. She is a 52-year-old business executive.

Patient: Doctor, I sometimes wonder if I've given you the wrong impression of myself. The Maxine Peroni we talk about here and the Maxine Peroni people at the office see are so different.

Therapist: How are they different?

Patient: The Maxine Peroni at the office is a self-confident, inventive, always-on-the-ball person who solves everybody's problems; she goes around saying that the time to solve a business difficulty, or any other kind of problem, is six months before it occurs. And, as we know, I'm not like that at all. I worry endlessly about everything, and getting out of bed every morning to go to the office is agony, thinking that this is the day I'll foul up everything. Someday the mask is going to fall off and that'll be the end of me.

Therapist: The mask? You've been a competent person in your work for almost thirty years now. It's unlikely that the role you play there is going to slip, let alone fall off. You've probably gotten continually better in your work as time has gone by; the problem is the distress that lies behind it. At home, in your marriage and with the two children you've reared, you've always been effective, and you've been much more comfortable there.

Patient: So what do we do?

Therapist: We look for answers. Why do the challenges of the job seem so much more threatening than those at home? More people probably fail on the home front than at work. You've succeeded comfortably where many people fail and also have succeeded, though uncomfortably, where most people tend to do reasonably well.

Patient: And which is the real me?

Therapist: They're both the real you. In talking about this we have outlined a new area to work on. Why is the job so threatening when realistically it ought not to be? What happened in the formative years of your life to make the world outside the home seem menacing while the world inside it was secure and at ease?

Patient: In some ways my dad was like I am. He used to say that . . .

The Role of Advice

The word advice has acquired a bad smell in psycho-therapy. To many psychotherapists it suggests giving sound counsel to people who because of their personality problems cannot accept it and act on it. "If I could do that sort of thing, Doctor, I wouldn't have to come to see you."

Ideally the patient, through extensive work on his problems in therapy, arrives at a point where he himself puts a desired course of action into words and then carries it out. However in some cases help from the therapist is necessary, and in giving this help the comments made in Chapter 1 on loaded questions and statements are relevant. In the following example a therapist employs a loaded question to give advice: "Since you now feel more secure and adequate, do you feel it's time to leave your current job, which is strong on long hours and weak on pay, and accept the Milligan Corporation's long-standing offer?" The therapist, in contrast, may do the same thing with a statement after therapeutic work has prepared the way: "You feel more secure and adequate as a result of the progress you've made in therapy and, as we long ago agreed, when this point arrived you would be ready to accept the Milligan Corporation's offer of a much better job than the one you have." Advice puts icing on the cake; baking the cake comes first.

There are two kinds of advice—advice to do something and advice not to do something. "I think a vacation right now would help you" falls in the first category, and "I think a vacation right now, with all the current changes and turmoil at work, would create more problems than it would solve" falls in the second category. From time to time a patient tells a therapist of a patently imprudent or even disastrous thing he or she has decided to do. At such a time we feel a therapist may give direct advice and he may sometimes do this even when the topic is relatively new and there has not yet been much work on it. "Mr. Collins, I don't think this is the time to borrow heavily on the assets of your company and go into a big expansion program that you will have to supervise. I don't think you're up to it right now." "Ms. Ribeiro, I don't think marrying Conrad is a good idea; you've known him for only three weeks. You have problems living with your parents, but we don't know enough about Conrad to know if you'd be better off with him." Such areas offer much material for psychotherapeutic work both in terms of the immediate situation and the patient's ways of handling any problems or opportunities that arise in his life.

When does a therapist call a patient's relatives to give advice, and how does he do it? "Ms. McDonald, this is Dr. Carter, Dick's psychotherapist. I feel it is my responsibility to call and tell you that I don't think that a man who is as depressed as Dick is should start out alone on a trip. He needs informed, caring people around him; he has them here and he won't have them on this trip. I told him this and I also told him I intended to call you and tell you the same thing." "Mr. Pulaski, I have some unpleasant information to give you; you should have it. Mrs. Pulaski has not been taking her antipsychotic medication for four weeks. I don't think she's being frank with you about this. If she continues not to take it there is about a seventy percent chance that within four to six months she will once more become very disturbed. In calling you I am going against her wishes and I'm breaking my confidential relationship with her; she did not want me to call you. It was a difficult decision. In the end I felt that this is the thing to do. This of course may end my therapy with her, but I hope not." Occasionally the problem is not to decide what is the correct thing to do; it is to decide what is the least incorrect thing to do.

Investigation of Abrupt Changes and Gaps in the Patient's Life Adjustment

When abrupt changes have occurred one or more times in a patient's life it often is useful to examine them in detail. Such changes may be unfavorable or favorable. In the second category, for example, why did the patient feel less tense and more worthwhile when she left home to attend college in a distant city? Was it because she was for the first time away from her parents and thus able to choose her friends rather than to live in social circles largely selected by her mother and father, and to make many other decisions on her own? Or was the patient's improvement because of something else that happened at the same time? Was it related to the collapse of her older sister's marriage and turbulent divorce? Her sister had long been held up to her as an ideal and the patient had been made to feel second-rate in comparison to her. Were still other relevant things going on at this time? What do all these things tell us about the way the patient was reared?

From time to time a therapist becomes aware that there is a gap in his knowledge of a patient's life history. In such cases therapeutic attention often has been so concentrated on certain aspects of the patient's life that some glaring omission was not noticed. Realization that such a gap exists may come either from something the patient says or during a systematic review of the case as the therapist reflects on it. For example, a therapist may suddenly become aware that there is a ten-year period in a middle-aged patient's early adult life about which nothing has been said. Investigation of it may reveal a period of cocaine usage and job instability. In another example a therapist may be chagrined to discover from a chance remark of the patient that his current marriage is not the only one in his life and that for several years in his twenties he had a marriage "that I could have done without." Examination of what went on in that marriage may be important. Sometimes there are simple explanations for such a gap. A patient may have worked abroad for several years in relative social isolation and in a culture different from his customary one; it was an important period vocationally but little of enduring emotional significance occurred. At other times the gap conceals a painful era of a patient's life and it is important to explore it.

In some cases a gap, when carefully investigated, turns out to have been a period of emotional illness. For example, periodic depressions, perhaps accompanied by alcohol abuse and lasting from six months to two years, may be the causes of gaps, especially when they were not diagnosed as psychiatric problems and were not treated. "I didn't do much during 1984 and the first half of 1985, and the same thing happened for a while in the early '90s; I just lay around the house and hit the bottle a lot." Hypomanic periods may be camouflaged similarly. "That was when for six months I got the big idea that I ought to go into politics; I registered as a candidate for mayor and rushed around buttonholing people and making speeches. Finally my wife and my friends talked me out of it. That's happened twice in my life. The other time I wanted to expand my store into a chain all across the state. My wife, my accountant, and the whole family were down on me like a ton of bricks and wouldn't let me do it. Finally I gave up." Such information may be important in long-term special counseling for a patient and his family.

The Threefold Nature of Each Person-to-Person Relationship

In doing psychotherapy it often is helpful to explore each interpersonal relationship and event in terms of *needs, developments,* and *expectations.* In each person-to-person event (a) the needs of each involved person are met or not met, (b) the ongoing relationship develops in healthy or unhealthy ways, and (c) each person forms expectations of fulfillment or non-fulfillment of his or her future needs.

Let us examine such needs, developments, and expectations in an event in a relatively simple relationship, that of a mother breast-feeding her child. The child is hungry (a need) and cries, evoking a loving response (the mother's need is to care for her child in an affectionate manner). During the breast-feeding the mother–child relationship develops in a healthy way, and both the infant and the mother form expectations that both their needs will in the future be met in a similarly healthy manner.

In contrast, another infant has a need for food and cries, but the mother, being tired and irritable, handles the child in a rough, impatient manner and talks harshly. On this occasion the mother–child relationship develops in an unhealthy way and each of them has anxious or disgusted expectations of what future events of this kind will be like. Over a long period of time the impacts on both of them will be determined by whether such behavior by the mother is typical or atypical.

In the following abridged dialogue we shall in a similar manner explore the needs, developments, and expectations in person-to-person events in adolescence.

Patient: It was about nine o'clock and I was getting ready to go out and meet Fran at Wortley's for a burger and a milk shake. Mom came barging in and blew up. She said I wasn't to use any of her perfume and none of her earrings, and to put down that lipstick. She went off the deep end and asked if I wanted to look like a tramp and smell like a whore on the make. Get that! With *her* perfume and lipsick and earrings! But I didn't think of saying that until later. I never do. But I did tell her that that was no way for a mother to talk to her daughter, and it isn't. And one thing led to another and we ended up shouting at each another and I ran out of the house crying and spoiled my make-up. That sort of thing goes on all the time. If I'm going to be accused night and day of being a tramp I might as well be one. There are enough guys around for it. And she goes through all my clothes, shoes and shoe boxes looking for drugs, and I've never touched the stuff, and I've told her that a thousand times, but it's like talking to the wall. I'll be 15 in April and I know what I'm doing. I know how to take care of myself. I wouldn't have sex with any guy who wanted to do it bareback, and one shot of coke is education, not vice. Half the kids I know have tried it once. Not too many go beyond that. But I can tell you one thing. From now on I tell my mother absolutely nothing. Any time I go out it'll be to the library to look something up for school. From now on I'm meeting no one nowhere, as far as she's concerned.

Therapist: On your own?

Patient: All the way.

Therapist: And that's all to the good?

Patient: Sure. Why not?

Therapist: Nothing more to learn?

Patient: A lot to learn, but I'll learn it on my own.

Therapist: No friendly adult to answer questions or be a sounding board?

Patient: No. My dad is all tied up in that business of his.

Therapist: In my line of work we're great believers in question answering and sounding boards.

Patient: Where do they hand out that stuff?

Therapist: Right here. I love to answer questions and I'm the greatest sounding board this side of the Hudson River. Try me out. If kids like you didn't use me in this way I'd be out of a job, and the unemployment situation is bad enough as it is.

Patient: Maybe I'll do that sometime.

Therapist: I'll never tell you what to do, or what not to do. Among other things, it doesn't work. But I'm great with statistics on coke, crack and sex, bareback or otherwise. The one who decides what to do is you.

Patient: What do you do when a guy says, "Nobody likes a girl who is cold and crosses her legs every time a guy looks at her. I didn't know you were like that."

Therapist: What about saying, "I'll be hot as hell for the right guy when he comes along, but when he does I don't want my cunt to be as big as the Holland Tunnel."

Patient: My God! I couldn't say a thing like that.

Therapist: It stops them dead in their tracks, or at least slows them down a lot, and after blasting them with that they can't try to throw you off balance by accusing you of being a prude. Shock therapy. It usually works. Think about it.

In her relationship with her mother this adolescent's needs are not being met, and their relationship threatens to develop into one in which most expectations are barren. In contrast, her needs are being met in her interchange with the therapist, and a relationship is being developed that has constructive expectations.

The concepts of needs, developments, and expectations are useful in the field of working with parents who rear a child who is mentally retarded. Psychiatric social workers in some settings devote much time to this field. There is one aspect of this subject that often is overlooked. Many years ago the Social Security Administration ruled that some mentally retarded individuals over the age of 18 were entitled to pensions as disabled adults. It became necessary to evaluate large numbers of these persons and we, serving as consultants to the Social Security Administration, evaluated about fifty of them. It gave us an unusual opportunity to see how needs, developments, and expectations had worked out and were still working out in the lives of this particular group of handicapped individuals.

Many of them, and some had I.Q.s as low as thirty-five and forty, were meeting many needs of their aged parents, who in their early lives had met their children's needs and had developed healthy expectations in them. The other adult children in these families had moved out of the home, and many were living in distant cities with families of their own. Had it not been for the continued constructive presence of the mentally retarded child in these parental homes they would have been emotionally desolate and interpersonally barren. The retarded adult did many kinds of simple household work such as washing and drying dishes, tidying the house, raking leaves, and so forth. They also accompanied their parents during shopping trips, social visits, church attendance, trips to doctors' offices and to medical laboratories for tests, and other places. Some of them, though quiet in manner, had such good social behavior that people who met them often were unaware of their handicap.

Some Broader Aspects of Problem-Oriented Psychotherapy

Problem-oriented psychotherapy, because it is based on careful observation of what goes on between people and not inside them, lends itself naturally to the study of social, political, economic, and cultural problems. It can serve as a tool for understanding and solving difficulties in these fields.

In contrast, psychological systems that speculate on what goes on inside people can be employed to study broader social problems only by hammering them into new shapes. Can the Jungian system, with its concentric mental circles, imbedded archetypes, and various forms of unconsciousness be easily applied to understanding economic injustice, generation gap estrangements, and the controversies of affirmative action? Are Freudian mental schemes well suited to explain why people traffic in cocaine and have ethnic prejudices? Do Pavlovian conditioned reflexes, no matter how they are extrapolated into learning and behavioral theories, help to understand the aspirations and trickeries of a species that deals in abstract ideas? Is not a psychological system derived from observations of person-to-person relationships, feelings, and spoken thoughts more relevant to understanding the complex group activities we label social, economic, and political?

The Involved, Unobserved Observer

In investigating broad social problems the involved sharer we discussed in Chapters 1 and 2 becomes the *involved, unobserved observer*. The best student of the activities and difficulties of large groups of people is such a person. When people know they are being observed they begin to act in altered ways; they may become solicitously cooperative, or evasive, or resistant, or hostile. They never are as they ordinarily are, and conclusions then based on observing them are to some extent, and often to a large degree, unsound.

Observation is not the same thing as study; a subject may be extensively studied without being observed. Karl Marx studied English and German industrial society by spending 6 hours each day for twenty years in the library of the British Museum and produced an analysis that, despite some astute conclusions, was in general calamitously wrong. Adam Smith, without frequenting factories, warehouses, managers' offices, and the back rooms of shops, examined the British economic system of his day and found it to be a smoothly working system that served everyone harmoniously and well. If he had actually entered a British factory (and there is no evidence that he ever did—it is as if the author of a book on surgical technique never set foot in a hospital), he would have been dismayed to see that most of the workers in his oft-cited, smoothly running, beneficent pin factory were pallid, ragged, sick children and adolescents who never left the premises and whose wages were paid once a week at the factory door to their hungry, destitute parents. In evaluating large groups of people there is no substitute for direct involved experience by unobserved observers. The observer must mix with the people he is investigating—work with them, play with them—and draw his conclusions from what he sees, hears, smells, and suffers, or enjoys, while doing so. Scholarly study is not enough.

The Open-Minded Observer

The best observer is the one who goes about his or her task with as few preconceptions as possible about what he expects to see. He works with the same dearth of speculations and theories that we described in Chapters 1 and 2 as being necessary for a psychotherapist. The failure to do this leads to errors both in understanding what one observes and in recommending measures to solve the social problems on which one is concentrating. Two examples, again using Marx and Adam Smith as well known writers on social and economic issues, make this clear. Marx began with the assumption (or at least the strong prejudice) that property owners and business managers were grasping egoists who were indifferent to the suffering they caused their employees and others, and that working-class persons, in contrast, were unselfish and socially caring. This was basic, though vaguely stated (he assumed that property ownership was morally corrupting), in his doctrine that each capitalistic state would inevitably collapse and would be replaced by a humanitarian "dictatorship of the proletariat," and that there then would be a gradual "withering away of the state" because government would no longer be necessary to hold selfishness in check. This doctrine led to the dictatorship of Joseph Stalin and the most controlling government the world has known. The tragedy of Marxism arises from the fact that it was based on erroneous psychological assumptions. This would have been avoided if Marx had been both the open-minded observer and the involved, unobserved observer that problem-oriented psychotherapy proposes.

The same is true of Adam Smith. He began with the assumption that a person who pursues his own economic interests automatically contributes to the general welfare of society, because he produces something that society needs, and hence that the best government is one that in no way interferes with what he saw as the smooth, self-regulating, beneficent nature of a bustling industrial and commercial system. He thus provided ammunition that was employed for almost a century and a half (and is still so utilized in some parts of the world) to prevent factory reform, child labor laws, labor union legislation, unemployment insurance (it encouraged the working classes to be idle), and other welfare programs. If he had been both the kind of open-minded observer and the involved, unobserved observer that problem-oriented psychotherapy proposes, world history probably would have been much different.

We have already commented on the scientific basis of problem-oriented psychotherapy's approach to social problems at the beginning of this discussion. One special feature, however, must be pointed out. In the physical sciences experiments may be set up in the laboratory, or advantage may be taken of the ones that nature periodically sets up. In scientific social studies the latter type of experiment prevails; society itself sets up the experiments that the observer uses to prove or disprove his theses. Examples make this clear. The first proof of the validity of Einstein's revolutionary theories came from observations in 1919 of the effects of a solar eclipse on the courses of light rays from stars. It was a repeatable experiment; it could be done every time a complete solar eclipse occurred. Similarly, in the social sciences Sir Karl Popper, now considered the foremost philosopher of scientific methodology since Francis Bacon, feels that Marx's scientific socialism (Marx called it that and sought to make it adhere to scientific criteria) meets the criteria of a set of scientific hypotheses. However, they have been proved false by actual experience; Marxism is hence a false science in the same sense that astrology and alchemy are false sciences. This experiment has had similar observed results in other Marxist states in the twentieth century.

In summary, problem-oriented psychotherapy, because it depends on close observation of what goes on among people, lends itself to the study of social and economic problems, in contrast to systems based on introspection and the analysis of nonobservable internal psychological processes.

The threefold nature of person-to-person relationships in problem-oriented psychotherapy can be applied in studies of social groups. Large groups of people also have needs, developments, and expectations in each of their evolving trends and movements. In every wave of socioeconomic change needs are either met or not met, and depending on how they are met societies develop in healthy or unhealthy ways and form their expectations of the future.

Let us apply this threefold concept to a current movement in America, the use of home computers for acquiring many kinds of information, keeping personal and family records, receiving and sending mail and other communications, shopping, entertainment, and many other things. Computers are of course valuable, and have few drawbacks, in many home functions as well as in business offices, industrial processes, schools, scientific laboratories, and many other situations. Like all vast social developments, however, they have disadvantages. For example, does entertainment by computer games enhance or decrease the richness of an individual's interpersonal life and meet his needs for vibrant interaction with people? Is a computer game, played by a sedentary person in front of a screen, even though it may involve others in distant places, as emotionally healthy as playing basketball or baseball with a neighborhood group? Is a great deal of stimulating, direct person-to-person activity necessary to develop the players' capacities for teamwork, cooperation, compromise, and other essential interpersonal needs? Are physical skills, such as expertness in throwing and catching balls and estimating distances in split seconds, increased in computer games as they are in intense participation sports?

Does the computer player develop intuitive skill in evaluating people and learning to employ both their strengths and shortcomings for the good of a team and himself, as he does on the playing field? And does time spent in front of a computer mold the ways in which a person's expectations are formed for harmonious or harmful future involvements with people in social and economic life?

There isn't time for everything. Today the average American child or adolescent spends a little more than 4 hours a day passively watching a television screen and not interacting with people. If computer proponents have their way, will several hours of computer time be added to this television time, or will one cut into the other? We have long heard that the most important thing in education consists of vital teacher–student give-and-take experiences; does that happen to some extent in computer education, or does it happen at all? Is time spent before an electronic screen, be it that of a computer or a television set, truly beneficial in meeting emotional needs in developing interpersonal capacities, and in molding healthy expectations of interpersonal living in future years?

A vast social change is occurring in America and crucial questions are not being sufficiently asked; in some sectors of society they are not being asked at all. Should problem-solving psychotherapy's concept of needs, developments, and expectations be employed to evaluate where we are going in this respect?

Examination of a Society's View of Itself

Scrutiny of a society's view of itself and comparison of that view with reality may be revealing. It may lead to healthy changes in how a society thinks and acts. We can talk of a social self-image in the same way that we can talk of an individual one and learn much from it. The differences between what a society thinks of itself and what the facts are may be striking. For example, we may consider the widespread American view that they are among the most generous people in the world toward less fortunate nations. A recent survey revealed that the American public estimates that between twenty and forty percent of the federal government's budget goes to foreign aid. The fact is that only a fraction of one percent of that budget is marked for such purposes. It is the lowest percentage among the major industrialized countries. The same general situation prevails in private giving and nongovernmental organizations. Should this be changed?

Since this is a book on psychotherapy and not on sociology and economics we shall go no further in discussing how the principles of problem-oriented psychotherapy can be usefully applied to the analysis of social problems and finding solutions or improvements for them. We shall merely point out that other principles that may be particularly useful in this regard are (a) making and testing hypotheses about social measures, (b) the concept of energy flows in social activities and relationships, (c) the concepts of distortions as applied to group behavior and attitudes, and (d) the exploration of a society's possible or probable future as a way of seeing what may be the results of its current trends.

10 Problem-Oriented Group Psychotherapy

The Basic Types of Group Psychotherapy

In one-to-one psychotherapy, as noted earlier, only one relationship is available for direct scrutiny—the one the patient has with the therapist—and only one set of life experiences, those of the patient, are examined. The situation in group psychotherapy is different. In a group containing, for example, four patients and a therapist each patient has four person-to-person relationships available for observation—his relationships with the other three patients and his relationship with the therapist. Still other kinds of relationships are exposed as patients, singly or in combinations, interact with other members of the group and with the therapist. In addition, four groups of life experiences are laid out before everyone.

There are three basic types of group psychotherapy: (a) *exploratory group psychotherapy* in which the interpersonal relationships and emotional life of each member are examined and the interactions in the group itself also are observed, (b) *inspirational group psychotherapy* in which a number of people, who as a rule have a common difficulty, band together in fellowship and mutual help to solve their problem; there frequently is a nonsectarian religious spirit at work in these groups and in some of them a forceful leader actively conducts the sessions, and (c) *existential group psychotherapy* in which the group members deal with problems about the meaning and purposes of their lives. "What am I doing with my life? Isn't there anything better than this?" Such people often have a certain amount of anxiety and depression, and their relationships with others may be troubled.

We shall present abridged excerpts from the sessions of an existential therapeutic group. It met twice each week for sessions of one and one half hours each. The sessions occurred at eight-thirty at night in a supplementary office the therapist had in his home so that patients with demanding jobs could attend without inconvenience. The patients— Betty, Chuck, Tina, and Matt—were all between 25 and 40 years of age and were university graduates; three were married. Each patient paid per week what he or she would have paid for one hour of individual therapy. Each shortened excerpt is given a title.

The Functions of St. Thomas More and His Two Wives

Chuck: Betty, you haven't said a word all this session.
Betty: I've been through the wringer this week. A guy I know committed suicide on Monday.
Chuck: Oh.
Tina: How did he do it?
Betty: Rammed his car into a buttress on a freeway at one hundred and fifty miles an hour at one a.m.
Tina: How do they know it was suicide?
Betty: The seat belt wasn't fastened, he was alone, and what

was he doing speeding at that time of night in a part of
town he never goes to—and he had to be at work at eight
the next morning.

Chuck: Why did he do it?

Betty: Why does anybody do it? Just fed up. Everything cancels out everything else, and in the end you've got zero on
the bottom line.

Tina: (to the therapist) It's always more complicated than that,
isn't it?

Therapist: Mental health workers sometimes debate whether
such a thing as rational suicide exists.

Betty: Rational?

Therapist: Suicide as the result of calm reasoning by someone
who is not particularly depressed.

Betty: Someone who just wants out?

Therapist: In a sense, yes.

Betty: The Catholic Church, to which I am supposed to be-
long, says, in this country at least, that suicide is always the
result of mental illness. That way they get a church burial.
The family feels better.

Chuck: Insurance companies don't see it that way. All their
policies have clauses that say no payment in case of suicide.

Betty: They're only interested in making money. I don't see
how they can prove it one way or another with this guy. Insurance companies stall and argue, and wait to see if the
family takes them to court, and then settle out of court to
keep it out of the newspapers. Publicity gives other people
ideas.

Tina: Was anything wrong in his life?

Betty: Not that I know of, not that anyone knows of. Divorced,
two kids with his ex. But who isn't divorced these days? No
money troubles. I went to the funeral.

Tina: Who were there?

Betty: Not many people. His ex came. Guilt or curiosity,
I guess. His folks live in Denver, and only his brother
was there. A couple of people from where he works came,

and a few others whom I didn't know. It rained. We talked about the weather. It was awful. At the cemetery, lots of mud. There was only one happy guy and he was in the box.

Matt: What makes you think he was happy?

Betty: Feeling no pain.

Matt: And no pleasure either. He was nuts.

Betty: Talking of pleasure, tell us how joyful your life is at this time of year. Do you spend your time working night and day making out other people's tax returns, and drinking black coffee to keep at it? Big shot accountant!

Tina: This is getting pretty bitter and morbid. Let's change the subject.

Chuck: Sure, we're interested in life, not in cashing in your chips for no special reason.

Tina: What do you say about it, Doc? Give us the therapeutic viewpoint.

Therapist: People like this who commit suicide, if he was as truly undepressed as Betty indicates, usually lack a scaffolding in life. They have no set of ideas, feelings, or activities which make life meaningful and pulsating. It's our mal du siècle—the sickness of our time.

Tina: Where do they sell these scaffoldings?

Therapist: Quite a few places. Churches, for example, but business is rather slow there these days.

Betty: Yeah, nobody believes in God anymore. If you ask them they say they do, but they don't.

Chuck: And you?

Betty: Yes, more or less.

Chuck: And in fairies at the bottom of the garden?

Matt: Science has done away with God. We know too much now to need that crutch.

Betty: I don't know about that. Science explains things only in a narrow way.

Matt: Narrow?

Betty: Science only tells *how* things happen. It never tells *why*. Like the big bang theory about the beginning of the universe, and the big crunch theory about how it's going to end in fifteen billion more years. Suppose that one day they get it all worked out, down to the last detail. Then some guy or gal asks, why did it have to happen at all? And why did it have to happen the way it did, so that one fine day we came along? And they don't have any answer to that. All they can say is that that's the way it was, and is.

Matt: That's playing with words.

Betty: What else do we have? Only them and the thoughts behind them.

Matt: And do you think that if this guy who rammed his car into the freeway buttress had gone around asking why, why, why, he wouldn't have done it?

Betty: Maybe not. If you're really interested in things life looks different.

Matt: And just who knows why, why, why?

Betty: The padres say they do.

Matt: Oh Lord!

Betty: Well, you asked me a question and I gave you an answer.

Matt: And do you go every Sunday to hear all these answers?

Betty: Only once in a while. It's nice to know that somebody's working on it, somewhere.

Matt: The plaster saint kind of church?

Betty: There are fewer of them than there used to be.

Matt: "Look here, Saint Whoever You Are, you get me a motorcycle and I'll see that you get one hell of a lot of candles burning at your feet." These are answers, I suppose?

Betty: It's not that way. The saints are models of what we're supposed to aim at. Halfway between us and Him, since none of us are quite up to that. A lot of the saints were practical people—lawyers, businessmen, church administrators, and all sorts of other people. St. Thomas More was married twice, had kids and said that just as a man should not buy a horse without seeing him with the saddle off he ought not to marry a woman until he's seen her without any clothes on.

Chuck: That's the saint for me!

Betty: I doubt this guy would have committed suicide if he'd been thinking about things like that. When you're trying to figure things out you want to stick around and see what comes of it all.

Chuck: What was the name of that saint who went around looking at naked girls?

Betty: St. Thomas More. But if he were alive today I think he'd be satisfied with white wet bikinis.

Murray Steiner's Mission

Tina: Why are you arriving so late? The session's half over.

Chuck: I ran into Murray Steiner at a bar and couldn't get away from him. We spent three hours arguing about communism, or scientific socialism, as he calls it. He says all this business in Russia and China is just a temporary falling away, and that they'll see the light in time. He's crazy.

Tina: How can he still believe in communism after all that's happened?

Chuck: He's crazy, like I said. A nice guy, but crazy.

Therapist: For some people Marxism functions emotionally as a secular religion.

Betty: A what?

Therapist: A secular religion, or a materialistic religion. That's a set of ideas which, though not truly a religion, acts as a religion emotionally in the lives of some people. It gives meaning, purpose, and direction to their lives.

Chuck: That's Murray Steiner all right. No matter what you say he just stands there in that bar smiling at you with that

"Forgive them, Father, they know not what do" look on his face.

Tina: I don't see how intelligent people can believe in such things when they've been proved false right in front of their faces.

Chuck: Oh, he's got an answer for everything. They deviated from scientific socialism and their historical mission, beginning with Lenin. What a pile of shit!

Therapist: It's a powerful pile of shit. Dedicated communists believe in history with a capital H, a creative force that determines everything and explains everything.

Chuck: Murray's big word is mission, and when he says it he sounds like a Salvation Army bell ringer. Our mission, he says, is to move forward with history for the betterment of man. He gets a faraway look in his eyes when he talks of man's future, and has a dreamy smile on his face.

Matt: A moron!

Chuck: A moron hell! Murray Steiner is some sort of genius. They've got something named after him. The Steiner principle, or the Steiner particle, or something.

Matt: How can a guy like that believe such crap?

Therapist: They believe in it because the alternative is to believe in nothing—and that way lies desolation. It's paradise in this world and the gospel according to St. Marx, as the saying goes.

Tina: Aren't we wasting time talking about Marxism? What has that got to do with my problems?

Therapist: I think that what Chuck is trying to say is that Murray Steiner has found a psychological solution for a question that may bother you, that may be relevant to your problems.

Tina: What question?

Therapist: What am I doing here on this planet and how am I to pass my seventy-odd years so that life is not just a meaningless drifting from one damned thing to another. It works for Murray Steiner.

Tina: So if we all became scientific socialists we wouldn't have to come here twice a week anymore?

Therapist: Perhaps. But it wouldn't work for you anymore than traditional religious beliefs do. Materialistic religions are powerful forces in the twentieth century—probably the most powerful ones the century has produced.

Chuck: How many are there?

Therapist: Quite a few.

Chuck: Like what?

Therapist: Science, for some people, functions emotionally as one. Art is another. James Joyce is a good example. He was reared a devout Catholic, lost his faith in his adolescence and put his life back together again by art. He states his aim clearly—to create the uncreated conscience of the race, or something like that—toward the end of his autobiography, *Portrait of the Artist as a Young Man*. A lot of people agree with him.

Betty: So that's what goes on in *Ulysses* and *Finnegan's Wake*?

Therapist: For Joyce and some others, yes.

Betty: For me *Finnegan's Wake* is just the ultimate in crossword puzzles.

Matt: If I may be impertinent, I'd like to mention another one of these materialistic religions.

Betty: Well?

Matt: Psychoanalysis. I know people who believe in that as much as Chuck's barroom buddy believes in communism. For them it's a way of life and explains everything. Salvation through introspection and the gospel according to St. Sigmund, to paraphrase the doc.

Tina: Psychoanalysis is no religion. It's a science, a medical subject.

Matt: It may be, but what we're talking about is how people use it, the role it plays in their lives. Look at Ruth Mayhew. You and Betty know her. My God! She'd stop you on a street corner to convert you.

Betty: Maybe that's why Freud was such an atheist, and Marx too. I guess they knew a competitor when they saw one.

Therapist: "You shall have no other gods before me."

Matt: Who said that?

Betty: It's in the Bible, you idiot! The Ten Commandments.

Matt: Oh, yeah.

Tandem Polygamy

Matt: I'm glad this session is coming to an end. Tomorrow I've got to get up bright and early and drive out to Lake Forest. Henry Wilcox is getting married again.

Tina: Good Lord! Who's he marrying this time?

Matt: Some gal he met at a roulette wheel in Las Vegas. All bust and bottom and no brains at all, and one third his age.

Chuck: I remember the last one, or one of them. She had hair that came out of a box hanging down all over her face. Arnold Chang said she made love with the aid of a Seeing Eye dog.

Tina: Henry Wilcox must be 65 if he's a day. Isn't he ever going to settle down?

Matt: No. With him sex is what life is all about. I've seen his bedroom. That's where you throw your coat when you go to one of his Christmas parties. The biggest damned bed I've ever seen, a round one, and the walls and ceiling are covered with mirrors.

Betty: I went to his last wedding. He even had fireworks. His sons were there, managers of a couple of his businesses. It was weird, weird I tell you. And Henry—fat, with teeth that go on talking when he stops, which isn't often. Still, I like the guy. He's never hurt anybody and he's filthy rich. He's always good for a touch. Too bad he can't settle down.

Tina: Sex isn't enough to be a way of life.

Matt: Says you. You don't know Henry Wilcox. He's like those Hottentots in Darkest Africa who worship statues of erect penises. And he's not the only one. Look at our culture—our TV, videos, books, photography, and everything else—sex, sex, sex.

Tina: It *is* too much.

Matt: Tell that to Henry Wilcox. It's entertaining to be with him after he's had a few drinks. He gives a blow-by-blow description of sex with each of his seven wives. Sometimes he can't remember the names of one or two of them or gets them mixed up with each other. Everybody nearly dies laughing, with Henry joining right in.

Therapist: There's something forced and false in such people —a sort of desperation to be merry, for fear of what would happen if that ever broke down.

Matt: It's beginning to break down with Henry. His son Terry tells me he often gets weepy and keeps asking if he's getting old. Terry doesn't know what to say.

Betty: Another solution that's coming apart at the seams.

Tina: I wouldn't mind being married to Mr. Wilcox for a year or so. The alimony I'd get would solve a lot of my problems.

Chuck: You're not the first one to think that. The women use him more than he uses them.

Matt: This wedding is going to be the living end. I'm participating in the arrangements; that's why I have to go out early and check everything. Champagne flowing like water, expensive remembrances for everyone and vows to love, honor, and cherish forever and ever, and how this time it's for real, and how this time he's finally found the woman he's always been looking for. It'll be nauseating.

Betty: Then why are you going and are all involved in making some of the arrangements?

Matt: We do his accounting, dearie. Half the people who will be there are on Henry's gravy train, one way or another.

Betty: Typical of our society—the free market economy in full swing. There must be something more in life than that.

Matt: I guess so. I'll think about it as I guzzle the French champagne and the exotic food and smell the flowers especially flown in from Nicaragua and Venezuela.

Tina: It's a circus.

Through a Door, Darkly

Chuck: Tina, you look all pooped out. You're not quite with us tonight.

Tina: I was up until four o'clock this morning talking with my kid brother through a closed door.

Chuck: Through a closed door?

Tina: Yeah. He locked himself into his room eight days ago and refuses to come out or to talk with anybody except me. He just sits in there and smokes pot. They shove a plate of food in once a day when he opens the door a little, and then he's got half the furniture in the room piled against the door.

Chuck: Only pot?

Tina: A good question. Mom can't find some of her jewelry and his motorbike is gone. I suspect he's pawned or sold everything he can lay his hands on, and that kind of money suggests he may be into coke and crack as well. Mom is worried sick about him. Norton, he's her damned husband, wanted to call in the police and have them break the door down, or rush him when they shove the food in, but they gave up that idea when I mentioned that if they find coke or crack in there it'll get pretty grim. Then they thought of hiring private detectives or some other goons to do the door smashing or door rushing, but that would require spending money, something Norton doesn't like to do, especially if the goons found coke and started talking about their duty as citizens to report it to the police and had to be paid off not to. So they're back to square one.

Matt: I take it you don't like Norton.

Tina: Nobody likes Norton. Mom dumped Dad to marry him, thinking she was getting into high society. From the Young Matrons Club to the Junior League in one easy jump. She didn't count on Tommy's reaction to it. It caved him in. He's 19 and he's been kicked out of three universities in the last year and a half.

Chuck: And you're supposed to pick up the pieces?

Tina: I'm the only one he'll talk to, and even that is through a closed door.

Chuck: What do you talk about until four in the morning?

Tina: Lots of things. Hedonism, for example.

Chuck: What's that?

Tina: The department of philosophy that says that all there is in life is seeking pleasure—having fun. There's nothing more. Common or elegant—sex on the run or abstract art and highbrow books.

Betty: Eat, drink, be merry, for tomorrow we die.

Matt: Falstaff!

Betty: No, you numbskull. St. Paul's letter to somebody, probably the Romans or the Corinthians.

Tina: Well, to come right down to it, what else *is* there? Not that pot and crack are the best kind of fun—the price is too high, health-wise and money-wise—but that's what we're all after, isn't it? Hedoism—either the lowbrow or highbrow kind, like I said. Booze or ballet. The most pleasure at the most reasonable price. I prefer golf, bourbon on the rocks, and handsome men. You've got to set limits on it.

Chuck: Is Tommy bright?

Tina: Too damned bright. He's read everything, and remembers it. When Mom mentioned having Dr. Armstrong—he's a Presbyterian heavyweight—come to see him, Tommy quoted Bertrand Russell. He said that somebody once asked Bertrand Russell what he was going to do when he finally came face to face with God, and Bertrand Russell replied, "I shall say to Him, 'God, you gave us insufficient evidence.' "

Therapist: Anyway, it's a hopeful sign that Tommy will talk to you, even though it's through a closed door. If this goes on until four in the morning I take it you cover a lot of ground.

Tina: We wander all over the map. Yesterday it started at eight, or so. He likes to talk to me. But he won't open the door. He's afraid that Norton will try to get in somehow or other. He's got Norton and Mom up a tree. They're terrified that people are going to discover what's going on in that elegant house on Winchester Road.

Therapist: Vengeance.

Tina: Exactly, and Tommy knows it and intends to milk it for all it's worth. He hates Norton. So do I.

Matt: What's wrong with Norton?

Tina: He's a liar, among other things. He promised Mom a lot more than he's delivered. They built that house and furnished it, no holds barred, with the money Mom got from Dad when she divorced him. And now it's all gone and they live on Norton's money, and he wants to know where every cent goes, and argue about it. And he's loaded.

Chuck: A controlling sort of guy.

Tina: You can say that again. The house is completely air conditioned but all the controls are in Norton and Mom's bedroom. Tommy sits there in his room in August with his overcoat on. The windows are the kind that can't be opened. In fact it's those air conditioning controls that caused Tommy to flip completely a couple of years ago. He went into their bedroom to lower or raise the thermostat for his part of the house and he saw a couple of sex manuals on the bedside table. He can't stand the idea of Mom having sex with Norton. He won't even mention his name; he calls him "the old goat" and "that satyr."

Chuck: What else does Tommy talk about?

Tina: You won't believe this. We ran hedonism into the ground and now he's onto John of the Cross and Theresa of Ávila.

Chuck: Good God!

Tina: Exactly. Tommy says he is now exploring mysticism, stripped of religion and with the occasional use of pot. He says pot is not a drug; it's a herb, much favored by those Indians, or Native Americans as we're now supposed to call them, who live in New Mexico or Arizona, or maybe they use something else. He says John of the Cross has the right idea, if you take the religion out of it—through darkness to light and universal love. Et cetera.

Chuck: Who exactly is this John of the Cross?

Tina: A Spanish monk who lived four or five hundred years ago. He apparently was pretty much kicked around by the ecclesiatical authorities when he was alive, but after he was dead they decided he was a saint. He seems to have been quite a writer. Anyway, he stirs up people like Tommy, at least when he's on pot part of the time.

Chuck: And what do your mother and Norton think about this business of John of the Cross?

Tina: Believe it or not, the first time I mentioned him Norton asked if he was a rock star. I could have clobbered the guy.

Chuck: And your mom?

Tina: She doesn't care who anybody is. All she wants is to get that door open and get at her darling boy. She even fights with Norton about Tommy—the only thing she ever bucks him on. Like I said, Tommy's got them where he wants them, and he knows it. And there's nothing I can do.

Betty: Maybe our therapist here should accompany you on one of these through the keyhole tête-à-têtes. Doctor, do you make house calls?

Therapist: Once in a while.

Betty: Do you have any suggestions for Tina?

Therapist: Only lame ones. This family should have gone to a child guidance clinic about fifteen years ago. However, Tommy has a few things going for him. If he's reading, and remembering, Bertrand Russell, St. John of the Cross, and

St. Theresa of Ávila in that room of his he must be fairly
free of pot, or anything else, a good deal of the time. Also,
if he's been there for eight days his supply of drugs probably has run out or is about to run out, and he seems to be
making no moves to get out and replenish his supply.
That's a good sign. A very good one. In addition Tommy in
a very remarkable way seems to know what his problem is.
He's gone bankrupt emotionally and intellectually at a
young age but he knows it and he's looking around for
ways to become solvent again. It's a bit wild to give an
opinion about a patient I've never seen, but in a vague sort
of way I'm optimistic about Tommy. Or maybe I'm just
vicariously enjoying his sweet revenge on a couple of parents who have failed him badly.

Tina: I thought therapists were not supposed to get carried
away by their feelings about patients, even proxy ones.

Therapist: We too have one foot of clay. But we know it and try
to keep it in mind.

Are all these topics legitimate fields for psychotherapy?
We think so. You do what the patients need.

11 Combining Psychotherapy and Medications: A Brief Orientation for Nonphysician Psychotherapists

This chapter is divided into two sections. The first is a general coverage of the use of medications in treating emotional disorders; it is designed to be a brief orientation for nonphysician psychotherapists. The second section is a glossary to inform nonphysician psychotherapists about the specific medications that some of their patients may at times be taking. Almost all the commonly used medications in this field are listed, first by trade (generic) name, because that is how patients usually refer to them, and secondly by chemical (pharmacological) name because they often are so indicated in books and journal articles. It is anticipated that some readers will use this glossary as a desktop reference source, to be referred to from time to time when a patient mentions a medication that he or she is taking.

Antipsychotic and Antianxiety Medications

Since the early 1950s antipsychotic medications (and there were no truly effective ones before then) have greatly improved the treatment of schizophrenia, severe depressions, and manic disorders. When first introduced these medications were called major tranquilizers, but the term antipsychotic medications is now almost invariably used. Often they are simply referred to in terms of their usage, as antidepressant drugs or medications for schizophrenia. There is a current trend to make the term antipsychotic medication synonymous with medication for the treatment of schizophrenia. In contrast, the term minor tranquilizer was at first utilized for antianxiety (anxiolytic) medications; they too are now often referred to by terms that link them to specific psychoneuroses or emotional symptoms, as in the term antianxiety itself. The words neuroleptic and anxiolytic are synonyms of antipsychotic and antianxiety, respectively, but they are employed mainly in comprehensive works on this subject.

These medications have changed schizophrenia from a grim disorder with a bad prognosis into a treatable one with a good prognosis if proper medications are started in the early months or even within a year or two of the onset of the illness. Even when pharmacological treatment begins after that a good outcome may be obtained in many cases. Severe depressions have been telescoped by antidepressant medications, also first introduced in the 1950s, from one or two years to six to eight weeks; electro-shock treatment, which was available from about 1940 onward, gives equivalent results but involves hospitalization and various risks. The treatment of manic and hypomanic episodes has been similarly improved by the introduction of lithium salts and other drugs for their therapy. All these medications were discovered by chance; pharmacological knowledge that permits targeted searches for medications is a relatively recent development. Chlorpromazine, the first antipsychotic drug, was initially used as a pre-anesthetic medication; its remarkable effects on schizophrenia were afterwards observed. The first antidepressants were being employed, with some success, to treat pulmonary tuberculosis when physicians noted that many depressed tubercular patients taking them had striking recoveries from their depressions. The effects of lithium on mania were first observed, largely by chance, by a physician in Australia. Pharmalogical explanations about why these drugs work came later and there is still much to be learned on this subject.

The situation regarding the neuroses and the personality disorders is much different. Since the early 1950s many new antianxiety medications have been introduced and have been widely employed, and some of them have been advocated for specific psychoneuroses such as panic states and phobias. However in our opinion they have not significantly altered the long-term courses and prognoses of these conditions. We feel that the treatment of panic reactions, anxiety states, obsessive and compulsive disorders, the fatigue states (neurasthenia and others), conversion reactions and dissociative states (hysteria), and body overconcern (hypochondriacal) states, as well as personality disorders such as passive and antisocial personality problems, is still psychological. Psychotherapy remains the main useful treatment for this vast group of disorders, although some writers on this subject would disagree with us. The senior author of this book entered psychiatry in the late 1940s and has seen the rises and declines of various pharmacological treatments for the neuroses and the personality disorders—with their claims, counter-claims, initial hopes and long-term disappointments—and has come to view with skepticism each new wave of assertions that some recently launched medication decidedly helps in the treatment of neuroses or personality disorders. At the time of this writing the recent past has seen a wave of claims that new medications can resolve severe anxiety states, panic reactions, and phobias, and in the immediate present still other medications are being hailed as curative or markedly ameliorative agents in the treatment of obsessions and compulsions. We feel that it is doubtful that as the first decade of the next century draws to a close these assertions will be found to have been justified.

Antianxiety medications can take the edge off anxiousness to a maximum of twenty five percent (using the somewhat artificial device of percentages for this purpose) in some of the neuroses in which overt anxiety is a major feature, and they can help some individuals with personality disorders if they are anxiety-ridden. Medications thus make some patients more comfortable while they are working on their difficulties in psychotherapy. They also can be used to give periodic but not prolonged relief to anxious people who reject psychotherapy, but in such cases they should be prescribed by a physician who knows his patient well and who carefully explains the medicine's limitations. The relief these medications give to many patients is less than the above stated twenty five percent and in some cases it is negligible. In many instances the physician's reassurances and authoritative manner may be more important than the pharmacological effects of the medicines; disentangling the two is often impossible. There is always the risk, however, that a patient so treated, having experienced some relief with an antianxiety drug, will go "pill-hopping" and "doctor-shopping" to "find the right medicine for my trouble." Patients who do this as a rule do not go on to engage in psychotherapy, which might offer them a much better chance of solving their problems. Many patients would be helped if family doctors and other physicians routinely said, "This medication will take the edge off your tension. Getting your life and all its hang-ups straightened out will help you much more. If you can't make progress on your own in doing that consider getting help from the people who do this work fulltime." This is much better than "here's a pill for your nervousness."

When a psychotherapist undertakes work with a patient who is taking an antipsychotic medication during the convalescent and rehabilitative phases of a schizophrenic, severe depressive, or manic disorder, he may face the task of convincing the patient to continue to take his antipsychotic medication for the full time necessary to reduce the chance of a relapse. The therapist must in many cases involve in this effort the patient's family or other close persons with whom the patient has daily contacts. These people can, with the patient's knowledge and, hopefully, his consent, be alerted to make sure he takes his medication regularly. They also should be informed of the early signs of a relapse if the patient's daily maintenance dose is too low or if he or she is surreptitiously not taking the drug. Patients may assert they are taking it when in fact they are secreting tablets in their mouths and later spitting them out; it is for this reason, among others, that some of these medications are available in liquid form, to be washed down with a small amount of water after taking them. Patients may resist taking medications because they feel they do not need them anymore or they may wish to be rid of bothersome side effects such as dry mouths, slight involuntary muscular movements, and other annoyances. The main psychotherapeutic work at such times is of course to help the patient reintegrate himself into his social and vocational life and to regain self-confidence after the often shattering experience of having "cracked up." Psychotherapy on long-term personality problems and emotional difficulties can proceed with patients who are motivated to engage in it.

In our opinion the question is as yet unsettled as to whether psychotherapy decreases the chance that a formerly psychotic person will during his lifetime have more depressive or manic episodes or that a former schizophrenic no longer on medication will in time relapse. The jury is still out on this question, and when the final verdict is in it may well be different for different groups of patients. Thus persons who tend to slip from depressive episodes into manic phases at short intervals, or have frequent depressions or manic attacks, may turn out to be different in this regard from those whose psychotic episodes are separated by years or decades of good adjustment. The long periods of time needed to make studies on this subject render them difficult and expensive, and often the mental health workers who begin them are no longer professionally active when the studies are nearing their end. An example makes this clear. We recall a patient who over a thirty-odd-year period had six manic psychoses at roughly five-year intervals; after the age of 60 she had no more psychotic illnesses. However her sister, who had been her mainstay through decades of intermittent illness, had the first manic illness of her life at the age of 63 and then remained well during twelve years more of our observation of this family.

We feel that psychotherapy with a well-motivated, formerly psychotic patient is justified, but the patient and his family should be aware that present knowledge indicates that psychotherapy is not a guarantee against further illness.

Clinical and Legal Problems in This Field

A nonphysician psychotherapist should be aware of some of the clinical and legal problems that prescribing therapists sometimes encounter. This is particularly so if the nonphysician psychotherapist is working with a patient who is taking antipsychotic medication prescribed by a psychiatrist. There are, in order of increasing seriousness, two types of clinical difficulties that may occur in these patients; there are other possible complications but they are much less common. These two groups of problems are extra-pyramidal syndromes (EPS) and tardive dyskinesia (TD). The most common EPS syndrome is identical in symptomatology to parkinsonism (Parkinson's disease, or paralysis agitans). The patient who is so affected has general muscular rigidity: tremors of the hands, head, and possibly other areas; and a shuffling gait with short, rapid steps and a forwardly inclined body. If this syndrome causes a patient to have a serious accident at home or at work, or while driving his car or operating a power mower, a lawsuit against the prescribing physician may occur. The patient may claim that he was not properly warned of such possibilities, or that the physician should have decreased the dosage, or prescribed effective antiparkinsonian drugs, or discontinued the medicine. The second most common type of EPS symptoms consists of abrupt convulsive jerks of the arms, legs, or body, which may result in accidents at home, at work, or at play. EPS symptoms almost always disappear after the causative medication is discontinued, but this may require from ten days to three or four weeks. EPS symptoms may be combated by antiparkinsonian drugs, but such control as a rule is only partial.

A more serious complication is tardive dyskinesia (TD). This consists of uncontrollable constant movements of the lips, mouth, and adjacent regions; similar movements of the limbs and body also may occur. TD as a rule occurs only after a person has been taking an antipsychotic medication for a number of years, but when it occurs it may be permanent; measures to control these movements usually are unsatisfactory. Persons who were not warned of this risk may go to court and win large settlements. Even if they know of this possibility they may claim that their physicians should have noted the earliest signs of TD and stopped the medication before TD developed fully.

The prescribing physician thus is in a difficult position. If he stops an antipsychotic medication his patient may become psychotic again, and if he continues it he may end up with a serious clinical problem with possible legal implications. If early in the treatment, to avoid legal problems, he explains all aspects of this situation to the patient and his family, he is unloading onto lay persons a decision that only an experienced medical specialist is equipped to make; some patients thus informed at once stop their medications and in time become psychotic again. There is no satisfactory answer for these problems at this time. It is a subject that should be jointly addressed by physicians, legislators, and groups representing the public. A new code or set of rules and definitions is needed. A nonphysician psychotherapist, when he is working with a patient in this kind of situation, can only advise his patient to follow the advice of the prescribing doctor. Decisions and risks remain in that quarter.

We shall mention only briefly the problems that may occur in patients receiving lithium salts for recurrent mania (unipolar disorder; this term is at times also used to designate recurring depressive episodes) or alternating manic and depressive episodes (bipolar disorder). Lithium replaces the sodium ion in body salt and it may build up to dangerous levels in the blood and tissues because of marked sweating, diarrhea, vomiting, and other factors, precipitating a metabolic crisis. Deaths have occurred when such patients did not receive prompt hospital care. Over long periods of time lithium may also cause thyroid damage, kidney impairment, and other dysfunctions. The possible dilemmas faced by the prescribing physician are obvious when a manic-depressive patient needs lithium to remain free of crippling mental illness.

The clinical situation regarding medications in the neuroses and in personality disorders complicated by anxiety is, as mentioned earlier, far different. The courses and prognoses of these conditions have not been altered significantly by the medications introduced in recent decades and, in our opinion, the nonphysician psychotherapist is depriving his patients of little, if anything at all, by not being able to give them these agents. This is particularly so in the long run. Any relief these medications give tends to decrease rapidly after the first few weeks or months of their usage; thereafter the help they afford is small or negligible. Dosages cannot be continually increased as their effectiveness diminishes because of the risks of physical or psychological dependence as well as the side effects that larger doses often produce. For these reasons we employ antianxiety medications little in our work.

Disulfiram Therapy

Any discussion of medications employed for emotional disorders should include a brief consideration of disulfiram (Antabuse) in the management of alcoholism. This medication was discovered in the late 1940s and has been widely used since then. It produces no symptoms unless a person who is taking a daily tablet of it drinks alcohol. If he or she drinks alcohol, within ten to fifteen minutes he or she begins to have a severe headache, a feeling of tightness in the chest, flushing of the face, a sensation of pounding heartbeat, marked anxiousness, nausea, and at times vomiting. This reaction peaks in from 30 minutes to an hour and is over after 2 hours, leaving the person weak and exhausted for a couple of hours more. Disulfiram thus is a chemical barrier to drinking alcohol and as such is useful in a small but significant percentage of alcoholics.

To benefit from disulfiram an alcoholic must have a strong desire to stop drinking; it acts as a chain link fence to keep him or her from drinking when he or she is tempted to do so. It does not take away the desire for alcohol; that must come in time from the patient himself. In our experience about one

out of every six alcoholics to whom we offer disulfiram treatment accepts it, but those who do accept it, as a rule, continue
to take it and remain abstinent. Although psychotherapy
follows in some cases most disulfiram patients feel they do
not need it once they are no longer drinking. In contrast,
patients who are forced by their families or employers into
disulfiram treatment rarely do well in it; they feel that others
are "railroading" them and soon they are taking their tablets
irregularly or not at all. In our personal administration of
this treatment we always insist that the medication is given
once a day by a relative who watches the person take it; we
explain, quite sincerely, that this is routine for this treatment
as we conduct it.

It should be mentioned that Alcoholics Anonymous, an
inspirational group therapy approach that began in 1935
and is run by its own members, can aid another small but
significant percentage of alcoholics to become abstinent.
These two approaches can betweem them help about twenty-
five percent of alcoholics. Their similarity lies in the fact
that both depend on a strong desire by the person to stop
drinking. Both should be considered in any particular case
because the results of psychotherapy for alcoholism as a rule
are disappointing.

Sleep-Inducing Medications

The terms sleep-inducing and hypnotic are interchange-
able in pharmacology. In general medical writing a term that
includes the word sleep, such as sleep-producing or sleep-
inducing, is more commonly employed; expressions such as
sleeping medication and sleeping pills are often used by lay-
men. In formal medical writing hypnotic tends to be used.
The word sedative is a broad general term employed to indi-

cate any medication that calms a person; because of its non-specificity it tends to be less and less used in medical writing as time goes by.

As a rule we prescribe sleeping medication only for people who are sleeping badly because of some clearly defined stress of limited duration. This includes things such as a severe illness or some other crisis in the family, the death of a close person, unusual financial worries, and difficult personal and vocational decisions. After thirty days, for unclear reasons, sleeping medications work less well. If the prescriber continues to give a sleep-producing medication longer he often ends up increasing the dosage progressively with the danger of both physical and psychological dependence.

A small percentage of people, perhaps ten percent, appear to require much less sleep than others. We have seen a number of such people, including one woman who all her adult life slept only three hours a night (her husband and an adolesent daughter confirmed this); the energy levels of such people during the day are unimpaired. This seems to be more common in elderly individuals. Another point should be mentioned. Some patients complain that they sleep little during each night, but when these patients are for any reason hospitalized or when their relatives or others check them various times during the night they are found to be sleeping well. The explanation in many such cases is as follows. The patient awakes briefly from several to many times each night and sleeps well the rest of the time. A person remembers only his waking experiences; he cannot remember what happens during sleep or estimate, without checking a clock, how long he has been asleep during a nighttime interval. Thus the patient remembers only the several or many brief times during the night when he was awake and he feels he was awake almost the entire night. This occurs in persons of all ages and is particularly common in old age. In evaluating complaints of sleeplessness this possibility should be kept in mind, especially when the patient is bright-eyed and alert and does not sleep during the day.

The Otto Barker Phenomenon

The psychological factor in the effect of a sleeping medication is the main one in many cases. Many years ago we were consulted by an attorney, whom we shall call Otto Barker, for sleeping difficulty as he prepared for a series of important court cases. We prescribed one of the common medications used for insomnia. He canceled his next appointment and we heard no more from him. About three years later, at ten o'clock at night, we received a telephone call from him. He said that he had that day returned from a professional trip to a distant city and had only a few minutes before discovered that he had left his sleeping medicine in his hotel room. He said that he would be unable to sleep without it and requested that we at once arrange for him to get a new supply from a drugstore that was still open. Astonished, we asked if he had been taking this medication all this time and how he had been getting prescriptions for it. "Doctor," he replied, "I never took it. I just put it on the bedside table and, knowing that it was there if I needed it, slept all right. I've done that every night since I saw you. But I left it in Cleveland and I know I'll not be able to sleep without it." We arranged the medication for him. Since then we at times have referred to the large psychological factor in sleeping medication as the Otto Barker phenomenon.

It is a common observation when seeing a patient in hospital work, or during a house call or in an emergency room, that an upset person falls asleep soon after receiving an oral sleeping medication, long before it has reached a high enough level in the blood to produce sleep. In other instances a patient receives an intramuscular (not an intravenous) injection of a sleeping medicine and drops off to sleep as the needle is being removed, when little of the drug is yet circulating in his body. These are variations of the Otto Barker phenomenon. A patient's feeling of confidence in the doctor or in the hospital setting he is in as well as the quality of the doctor–patient or hospital–patient relationship is important in this regard.

Marx Therapy

When one of the authors of this book was a psychiatric resident physician he noted that during certain weeks when he was on night call he did not receive any calls from the ward nurse for orders for special or extra sleeping medication; during other weeks there usually were several such calls each night. In time it became clear that these weeks were the ones during which an elderly psychiatric nurse named Mrs. Marx (this actually was her name) was on night duty. We went to the ward one night to find out what occurred at these times. Mrs. Marx explained that when a patient couldn't sleep she went to the kitchen and prepared a large glass of warm milk with two teaspoons of sugar in it. She then gave the patient this milk and two standard-sized adult aspirin tablets, assuring the patient that he would soon be asleep (ward rules permitted the administration of small amounts of aspirin without a doctor's order). Aspirin, acetylsalicylic acid, after a brief excitatory effect on the central nervous system, exerts a certain sedative influence; milk protects the stomach from any irritative effects of aspirin. This usually worked, she said, but if it didn't she repeated the procedure once or twice and then it invariably did so. Calling this Marx therapy, we have employed it liberally on both outpatient and hospitalized patients for many years. The measures of our Mrs. Marx are much more effective than those of the well-known economist of the same name in another field.

A Glossary of Medications Commonly Used in Psychiatric Disorders

As we have noted, clinical psychologists, psychiatric social workers, and other nonphysician psychotherapists from time to time see patients who are taking medications that have been psychiatrically prescribed and it is useful for them to know something about these medications. A glossary of almost all the medications employed for psychiatric disorders follows. The trade (brand) name of the medication is first given because patients usually refer to it in this way. The chemical (pharmacological) name then follows in parentheses and after that the disorder or disorders for which the drug is utilized is indicated. When a medication is marketed under more than one trade name, information is given only under the trade name that comes first alphabetically; the reader is referred to that entry when subsequent trade names occur. Various other kinds of information are sometimes added when it is felt that it might be of help or interest to nonphysician psychotherapists.

At the end of the glossary all its entries are relisted alphabetically by their chemical names, with the trade name or names following. In many books and journal articles only the chemical names of medications are used; the editors and authors thus avoid giving gratuitous advertising to the trade names of medications, which are the sole property of the manufacturers.

There are three special entries in this glossary; they are on addiction, barbiturates, and non-antidepressant uses of antidepressant medications.

Adapin (doxepin). An antidepressant medication. It has been particularly recommended when anxiety is prominent in a depressive disorder. See entry under non-antidepressant uses of antidepressant medications.

Addiction. Physical addiction, or physical dependence, may occur when a person takes much more than the prescribed amount for about thirty days or more of any of the barbiturates (Nembutal, Seconal, and others), or any of the antianxiety medications (Librium, Valium, and others), or any of the sleep-inducing medications (Ambien, Halcion, and others). The degree of physical dependence and the severity of withdrawal symptoms upon abrupt cessation depend mainly on the amount the person has been taking, but other factors also may be important. Physical addiction does not occur with any of the antipsychotic medications (Thorazine, Elavil, Eskalith, and others) employed in the treatment of schizophrenia, depression, and mania, regardless of the dosage and the length of time the drug is taken. Psychological addiction, or psychological dependence, can occur with any of the barbiturates or antianxiety and sleep-inducing medications, but it is rare with any of the antipsychotic medications.

Ambien (zolpidem). A sleep-inducing medication.

Antabuse (disulfiram). A medication used in the treatment of alcoholism. See the discussion of disulfiram therapy in this chapter.

Artane (trihexiphenidyl). A medication employed to decrease the parkinsonian symptoms (described earlier in this chapter) that may occur as side effects of many drugs utilized in the treatment of schizophrenia. This medication, plus others [Benadryl, Cogentin, Inderol, Kemadrin and Tremin (which chemically is the same as Artane)] listed in this glossary, are so commonly used for this purpose in schizophrenic patients that a nonphysician psychotherapist should understand their significance when he or she encounters a patient who is taking one of them in conjunction with an antipsychotic drug.

Asendin (amoxapine). An antidepressant medication. See entry under non-antidepressant uses of antidepressant medications.

Ativan (lorazepam). An antianxiety medication. Ativan belongs to the chemical group of the benzodiazepines

(Librium, Valium, and others); these medications are occasionally used as mild sleep-inducing drugs, muscle relaxants, and adjuncts to anticonvulsive (anti-epileptic) drugs, some being favored for one or more of these purposes.

Aventyl (nortriptyline). An antidepressant medication. See entry under non-antidepressant uses of antidepressant medications.

Barbiturates, general notation. The barbiturates (Nembutal, Seconal, and others) are much less prescribed today than formerly because (a) the daily dosage which causes physical dependence, or addiction, is closer to the daily dosage employed therapeutically than is the case with the drugs introduced since the 1950s for daytime anxiousness (Librium, Valium, and others) and the more recently introduced sleep-inducing medications (Ambien, Halcion, and others), and (b) the amount which is likely to prove fatal in a suicidal attempt is lower with barbiturates than with any other group of calming medications, such as nonbarbiturate antianxiety agents, nonbarbiturate sleep-inducing drugs and the antipsychotic medications. The main exception is Luminal (phenobarbital), which worldwide is still a mainstay in the treatment of epilepsy. Some barbiturates are used for preanesthetic, preelectroshock, and other special purposes.

Benadryl (diphenhydramine). An antiparkinsonian medication. See entry under Artane. In general medical work Benadryl is mainly prescribed, however, for allergic and allied conditions.

Clozaril (clozapine). An antipsychotic medication often used in treating schizophrenics who have proved refractory to other drugs; it affects negative symptoms of schizophrenia such as withdrawal and blunting of affect, as well as positive symptoms such as hallucinations and delusions. Patients receiving it must be closely followed because in a small percentage of cases severe adverse blood reactions occur. Despite this shortcoming some clinicians feel it now is the drug of choice for most cases of schizophrenia.

Cogentin (benztropine). An antiparkinsonian medication. See entry under Artane.

Cylert (pemoline). A medication sometimes used in treating attention deficit disorder (ADD). See entry under Ritalin.

Dalmane (flurazepam). A sleep-inducing medication. See entry under Ativan.

Depakene (valproate). An anticonvulsive medication that is also sometimes used in treating manic disorders. See entry under Tegretol.

Depakote (divalproex). A recently introduced medication for the treatment of manic episodes.

Desyrel (trazodone). An antidepressant drug. It is more sedating than some other antidepressants and hence some clinicians employ it in depressed patients who also are anxious or agitated. See entry under non-antidepressant uses of antidepressant medications.

Effexor (venlafaxine). An antidepressant medication. Some studies suggest special utility in cases of depression in which anxiousness is a prominent feature. See entry under non-antidepressant uses of antidepressant medications.

Elavil (amitriptyline). An antidepressant medication. See entry under non-antidepressant uses of antidepressant medications.

Endep (amitriptyline). See entry under Elavil.

Equanil (meprobamate). An agent used for daytime anxiousness and, in larger doses, for sleep-induction; it is also prescribed as a muscle relaxant. Meprobamate, under the trade name Miltown, was in the 1950s the first of the new nonbarbiturate antianxiety drugs to attract wide attention in the lay press.

Eskalith (lithium carbonate). A medication employed in the treatment of mania. See discussion in a preceding section of this chapter.

Halcion (triazolam). A sleep-inducing medication. See entry under Ativan.

Haldol (haloperidol). An antipsychotic medication used mainly in the treatment of schizophrenia. It is also available in a preparation for slow absorbing intramuscular depot injection; in this form it is given about once a month in most cases, although schedules differ from patient to patient. Haldol is now also the most used drug for alleviating the multiple severe tics and other symptoms of Gilles de la Tourette's syndrome, a disorder that begins in childhood, affects boys much more than girls, and characteristically is lifelong. Prozac and other medications are likewise at times employed in Tourette's syndrome, the concept of which has been somewhat enlarged in recent years to include some patients with severe obsessions coupled with marked compulsive gestures and acts.

Inderol (propanolol). An antiparkinsonian medication. See entry under Artane.

Kemadrin (procyclidine). An antiparkinsonian drug. See entry under Artane.

Klonopin (clonazepam). An antianxiety medication. See entry under Ativan.

Librium (chlordiazepoxide). An antianxiety medication. See entry under Ativan.

Lithane (lithium carbonate). See entry under Eskalith.

Lithobid (lithium carbonate). See entry under Eskalith.

Lithonate (lithium carbonate). See entry under Eskalith.

Loxitane (loxapine). An antipsychotic drug employed mainly in the treatment of schizophrenia.

Ludiomil (maprotiline). An antidepressant drug. See entry under non-antidepressant uses of antidepressant medications.

Luminal (phenobarbital). A slow acting barbiturate with a long period of activity. See entry under barbiturates, general notation.

Luvox (fluvoxamine). A medication recently introduced for the treatment of obsessive-compulsive neuroses.

Mellaril (thioridazine). An antipsychotic medication used mainly in treating schizophrenia.

Miltown (meprobamate). See entry under Equanil.

Mobam (molindone). An antipsychotic medication employed chiefly in the treatment of schizophrenia.

Nardil (phenelzine). An antidepressant medication. If patients on this medication ingest beer, wine, cheese, or some other foods, crises of high blood pressure may occur with severe headaches, various other symptoms and, occasionally, intracranial bleeding. In the popular press it has been called "the cheese drug." See entry under non-antidepressant uses of antidepressant medications.

Navane (thiothixine). An antipsychotic agent used mostly in treating schizophrenia.

Nembutal (pentobarbital). A quick acting barbiturate with a duration of action of moderate length. See entry under barbiturates, general notation.

Noctec (chloral hydrate). A long-established sleep-inducing medication available both in liquid form and in capsules. In older novels and short stories it is occasionally mentioned as "chloral drops," and the "Mickey Finns" and "Mickeys" of early crime and detective fiction consisted of chloral hydrate in alcoholic beverages.

Non-antidepressant uses of antidepressant medications. Antidepressant drugs have been reported to be useful in some cases of (a) obsessive-compulsive neuroses, especially Prozac, (b) panic states, (c) severe phobias, (d) enuresis in children and adolescents, as opposed to elderly patients, especially Presamine, or Tofranil, (e) excessive sleepiness and some other sleep disturbances, (f) compulsive episodic overeating (bulimia), (g) cocaine addiction, chiefly Norpramin, or Pertofrane, (h) narcolepsy, a disorder characterized by sudden attacks of sleepiness (as in the fat boy in Dickens's *The Pickwick Papers*) or by episodes of abrupt loss of muscle tone, (i) occasional cases of refractory schizophrenia, as an adjunct to antipsychotic medications, (j) migraine and some other pain syndromes, and (k) attention deficit disorder (ADD) in children. In some of these disorders, as in the use of Presamine, or Tofranail, in enuresis, their utility is well established, but many clinicians feel that much more evaluation is needed before their statuses in some of these other difficulties are clear.

Norpramin (desipramine). An antidepressant medication. See entry under non-antidepressant uses of antidepressant medications.

Parnate (tranylcypromine). An antidepressant agent. It is subject to the same dietary precautions as Nardil. See entry under Nardil. See entry under non-antidepressant uses of antidepressant medications.

Paxil (paroxetine). An antidepressant medication. Some studies suggest that it reduces anxiousness in an agitated depressed patient. See entry under non-antidepressant uses of antidepressant medications.

Paxipam (halazepam). An antianxiety medication. See entry under Ativan.

Permitil (fluphenazine). An antipsychotic medication employed chiefly in treating schizophrenia. Fluphenazine is available in a long-acting depot intramuscular injection preparation under the trade name Prolixin (but not under its alternate trade name Permitil). See entry under Haldol, which is also available for depot intramuscular injection.

Pertofrane (desipramine). See entry under Norpramin.

Presamine (imipramine). An antidepressant medication. Imipramine, most often under the alternate trade name Tofranil, is much used in the treatment of enuresis in children and adolescents. Small nighttime doses eliminate this symptom in about two thirds of cases, but more than one period of utilization may be needed before final control is achieved. Imipramine exerts this effect by virtue of its tendency to dampen the muscles involved in emptying the bladder. See entry under non-antidepressant uses of antidepressant medications.

Prolixin (fluphenazine). See entry under Permitil.

Prozac (fluoxetine). An antidepressant medication that since its relatively recent introduction has been widely used. However, there have been problems associated with it, including much litigation; about one hundred and sixty lawsuits are pending against its manufacturer at the time of this writing. The most common allegation is that it produces psychomotor agitation as one of its occasional side effects and may thus precipitate suicide and violent attacks on others. See entry under non-antidepressant uses of antidepressant medications.

Restoril (temazepam). An antianxiety medication. See entry under Ativan.

Revia (naltrexone). A drug marketed recently under this trade name as an adjunct in the treatment of alcoholism. It has for a number of years been available under the trade name Trexcin as an aid in treating narcotic addiction.

Risperdal (risperidone). A recently introduced antipsychotic medication for the treatment of schizophrenia. It is related in general nature and action to Clozaril.

Ritalin (methylphenidate). The main medication employed in the treatment of attention deficit disorder (ADD). Though useful in the management of the hyperactivity and distractibility of children with this difficulty, many clinicians feel that its long-term benefit, in terms of adjustment in adolescence and adulthood, has not been conclusively demonstrated.

Seconal (secobarbital). A quick acting barbiturate with a short duration of action. It is sometimes employed for preanesthetic, preoperative and similar purposes. See entry under barbiturates, general notation.

Serax (oxazepam). An antianxiety medication. See entry under Ativan.

Serontil (mesoridazine). An antipsychotic agent employed chiefly in the treatment of schizophrenia.

Serzone (nefazodone). A recently released antidepressant medication. See entry under non-antidepressant uses of antidepressant medications.

Sinequan (doxepin). See entry under Adapin.

Sparine (promazine). A mild antipsychotic medication now employed mainly in assuaging agitation in patients with senility (Alzheimer's disease or senile cerebrovascular disorders) and other organic brain diseases.

Stelazine (trifluoperazine). An antipsychotic medication mostly utilized in treating schizophrenia.

Surmontil (trimipramine). An antidepressant medication. See entry under non-antidepressant uses of antidepressant medications.

Tegretol (carbamazine). A medication mainly used in the treatment of epilepsy. However it occasionally is employed in cases of mania (unipolar disorder) and manic-depressive (bipolar) disorder when lithium treatment is for any reason unworkable or inadvisable. It tends to be given to patients whose episodes of mood disturbance occur at close intervals.

Thorazine (chlorpromazine). An antipsychotic medication employed chiefly in the treatment of schizophrenia. Chlorpromazine was the first antipsychotic medication to be introduced in the early 1950s, and on a worldwide basis is probably still the most used drug for schizophrenia. This is because (a) the patent on it has expired (after which time only trade names for a drug can be registered as the exclusive property of manufacturers), and hence any commercial, governmental, or philanthropic organization can produce and distribute it, (b) it is relatively inexpensive and easy to manufacture, (c) its short-term and long-term side effects are well understood and ways for dealing with them or avoiding them are standard knowledge, and (d) some clinicians feel that no subsequently released medication for the treatment of schizophrenia over long periods of time is truly superior to it.

Tofranil (imipramine). See entry under Presamine.

Tremin (trihexiphenidyl). See entry under Artane.

Valium (diazepam). An antianxiety medication. See entry under Ativan.

Vesprin (trifluopromazine). An antipsychotic medication used mainly in the treatment of schizophrenia.

Vivactil (protriptyline). An antidepressant medication. See entry under non-antidepressant uses of antidepressant medications.

Wellbutrin (bupropion). An antidepressant medication. See entry under non-antidepressant uses of antidepressant medications.

Xanax (alprazolam). An antianxiety medication. See entry under Ativan.

Zoloft (sertraline). An antidepressant medication. See entry under non-antidepressant uses of antidepressant medications.

In reading psychiatric books and journal articles, as briefly noted at the beginning of this section, a therapist may find a medication mentioned only by its chemical name. This is preferred by many professional journals and book publishers because it does not give publicity to the trade name, which is the exclusive property of the pharmaceutical manufacturer. Hence each medication of this glossary is below listed alphabetically by its chemical name with the trade (brand) name following it. In some cases a medication is marketed under more than one trade name; some medications therefore have two, and in one case four, trade names listed after them.

alprazolam (Xanax).
amitriptyline (Elavil, Endep).
amoxapine (Asendin).
benztropine (Cogentin).
bupropion (Wellbutrin).
carbamazine (Tegretol).
chloralhydrate (Noctec).
chlordiazepoxide (Librium).
chlorpromazine (Thorazine).
clonazepam (Klonopin).
clozapine (Clozaril).
diazepam (Valium).
diphenhydramine (Benadryl).
disulfiram (Antabuse).
divalproex (Depakote).
doxepin (Adapin, Sinequan).
fluoxetine (Prozac).
fluphenazine (Permitil, Prolixin)
flurazepam (Dalmane).
fluvoxamine (Luvox).
halazepam (Paxipam).
haloperidol (Haldol).
imipramine (Presamine, Tofranil).
lithium carbonate (Eskalith, Lithane, Lithobid, Lithonate).
lorazepam (Ativan).
loxapine (Loxitane).
maprotiline (Ludiomil).
meprobamate (Equanil, Miltown).
mesoridazine (Serontil).
methylphenidate (Ritalin).
molindone (Mobam).
naltrexone (Revia).
nefazodone (Serzone).
nortriptyline (Aventyl).
oxazepam (Serax).

paroxetine (Paxil).
pemoline (Cylert).
pentobarbital (Nembutal).
phenelzine (Nardil).
phenobarbital (Luminal).
procyclidine (Kemadrin).
promazine (Sparine).
propranolol (Inderol).
protriptyline (Vivactil).
risperidone (Risperdal).
secobarbital (Seconal).
sertraline (Zoloft).
temazepam (Restoril).
thioridazine (Mellaril).
thiothixine (Navane).
tranylcypromine (Parnate).
trazodone (Desyrel).
triazolam (Halcion).
trifluoperazine (Stelazine).
triflupromazine (Vesprin).
trihexiphenidyl (Artane, Tremin).
trimipramine (Surmontil).
valproate (Depakene).
venlafaxine (Effexor).
zolpidem (Ambien).

References

Altshuler, K. Z. (1989). Will the psychotherapies yield differential results? A look at assumptions in therapy trials. *American Journal of Psychotherapy* 43:310–320.

Basch, M. F. (1992). *Practicing Psychotherapy: A Casebook.* New York: Basic Books.

Beck, A., Wright, F. D., Newman, C. P., and Leise, B. S. (1993). *Cognitive Therapy of Substance Abuse.* New York: Guilford.

Bergin, A. E., and Garfield, S. L. (1994). *Handbook of Psychotherapy and Behavior Change,* 4th ed. New York: John Wiley and Sons.

Bloch, S., Hafner, J., Herari, E., and Szmukler, G. I. (1994). *The Family in Clinical Psychiatry.* New York: Oxford University Press.

Bongar, B., and Beutler, L. E., eds. (1994). *Comprehensive Textbook of Psychotherapy: Theory and Practice.* New York: Oxford University Press.

Budman, S. H., Hoyt, M. F., and Friedman, S. (1992). *The First Session in Brief Psychotherapy*. New York: Guilford.

Cavaley, R. H. (1993). Psychiatry is more than a science. *British Journal of Psychiatry* 162:154–160.

Chapman, A. H. (1978). *The Treatment Techniques of Harry Stack Sullivan*. New York: Brunner/Mazel. (1996) Northvale, NJ: Jason Aronson, Master Work Series.

Chapman, A. H., and Chapman-Santana, M. (1994). Is it possible to have an unconscious thought? *The Lancet* 344: 1752–1753.

Chapman, A. H., and Santana, M. C. M. (1980). *Harry Stack Sullivan's Concepts of Personality Development and Psychiatric Illness*. New York: Brunner/Mazel.

Heather, N. (1989). Psychology and brief interventions. *British Journal of Addiction* 84:357–370.

Heim, E., Blaser, A., Ringer, C., and Thommen, M. (1990). Overview of brief psychotherapies—a basis for discussion of problem oriented therapy. *Psychotherapy Psychosomatic Medicine and Psychology* 40:158–164.

Horowitz, L. M., Rosenberg, S. E., and Bartholomew, K. (1993). Interpersonal problems, attachment styles, and outcome in brief dynamic psychotherapy. *Journal of Consulting and Clinical Psychology* 60:549–560.

Isometon, E. T., Heikkinen, M. E., Marttunen, M. J., et al. (1995). The last appointment before suicide: Is suicide intent communicated? *American Journal of Psychiatry* 152:919–922.

James, I. A., and Blackburn, I. M. (1995). Cognitive therapy with obsessive compulsive disorder. *British Journal of Psychiatry* 166:444–450.

Keitner, G. I., Miller, I. W., and Ryan, C. E. (1993). The role of the family in major depressive illness. *Psychiatric Annals* 23:500–507.

Luborsky, L., Barber, J., and Crits-Cristoph, P. (1990). Therapy-based research for understanding the process of dynamic psychotherapy. *Journal of Consulting and Clinical Psychology* 58:281–287.

Morrison, J. (1994). *The First Interview*. New York: Guilford.

Reich, J. H., and Green, A. I. (1990). Effect of personality on outcome of treatment. *Journal of Nervous and Mental Disease* 178:592–600.

Ringer, C., Blaser, A., Thommen, M., and Heim, E. (1990). Problem oriented therapy. A new therapeutic and didactic concept. *Psychotherapy Psychosomatic Medicine and Psychology* 40:165–171.

Saretsky, T. (1994). *Active Techniques and Group Psychotherapy*. Northvale, NJ: Jason Aronson.

Schachter, M. (1994). *Psychotherapy and Medication*. Northvale, NJ: Jason Aronson.

Schwartz, H. J., Bleiberg, E., and Weissman, S. (1995). *Psychodynamic Concepts in General Psychiatry*. Washington, DC: American Psychiatric Press.

Screiber, J. C., Brier, A., and Pickar, D. (1995). Expressed emotion. Trait or state? *British Journal of Psychiatry* 166:647–650.

Shanks, M. F., and Ho-Yen, D. O. (1995). A clinical study of chronic fatigue syndrome. *British Journal of Psychiatry* 166:
798–801.

Spiro, H., Curnen, M. G. M., Reschel, E., and St. James, D. (1993). *Empathy and the Practice of Medicine*. New Haven, CT: Yale University Press.

Strupp, H. H. (1993). The Vanderbilt studies: synopsis. *Journal of Consulting and Clinical Psychology* 61:431–433.

Strupp, H. H., Hadley, S. W., and Gomes-Schwartz, B. (1994). *When Things Get Worse: The Problem of Negative Effects in Psychotherapy*. Northvale, NJ: Jason Aronson.

Thommen, M., Blaser, A., Binger, C., and Heim, E. (1990). The value of subjective illness theories in problem oriented therapy. *Psychotherapy Psychosomatic Medicine and Psychology* 40:172–177.

Tuyn, L. K. (1992). Solution-oriented therapy and Rogerian nursing science: an integrated approach. *Archives of Psychiatric Nursing* 6:83–89.

Winer, R. (1994). *Close Encounters: A Relational View of the Therapeutic Process.* Northvale, NJ: Jason Aronson.

Index

Addictions, 130
    alcohol, 189–190, 201
    narcotic, 199, 201
Administrative reasons, for
    therapy, 109–111
Adolescents, 201
    examples of work with,
        135–136, 154–156
    families' deterring therapy
        of, 129–130
Advice, from therapist,
    77, 145–146,
    150–151
Alcoholism, 189–190, 201
Antabuse, to treat alcoholism,
    189–190
Antianxiety medications,
    182–186, 188–189
    glossary of, 194–205
Antidepressants, glossary of,
    194–205

Antipsychotic medications,
    182–189
    glossary of, 194–205
Anxiety, 18, 23
    and antianxiety
        medications, 182–186,
        188–189, 194–205
    blocking communication,
        40–42
    methods of reducing, 15,
        42–45, 136–137
Assimilation, of experiences,
    29–32, 36
    pain as obstacle to,
        45–48
Attacks on therapist, as
    unhealthy well-being
    operation, 69–70
Attention deficit disorder
    (ADD), medications for,
    199–201

Behavior, therapist's, 109, 111–118. *See also* Observable behaviors

Blanket agreement, as unhealthy well-being operation, 67–69

Certification boards, 115–116

Changes, in patient's life, 152–153

Characterological problems, 101–103, 105–107

Children, 201
as patients, 75–76, 109, 129–130

Communication. *See also* Nonverbal communication
deteriorating in therapy, 125–130
pain as hindrance to, 39–45

Compensatory reactions, as well-being operation, 61

Computers, analysis of effects of, 161–163

Confidentiality, breaking, 151

Data. *See* History

Daydreams, 53–54

Denial, as unhealthy well-being operation, 64–65

Depression, 87
medications for, 182–186, 194–205

Deteriorating communication, in therapy, 125–130

Deviations in therapy, 109–111

Direction, by therapist, 10–13, 141–146

Distortions, 101–120

Disulfiram (Antabuse), to treat alcoholism, 189–190

Dreams, 48
not used in problem-oriented psychotherapy, 130–134

Drugs. *See also* Medications
abuse, 130
discussion in groups, 175–176, 178–179

Emotions, 15–16. *See also* Pain
blocking therapy, 16, 19, 67, 125–130
and nonperception, 21–24
sublimation of, 59–60
therapist's, 1, 52, 112–114

Energy flows, in relationships, 90–100

Enuresis, medications for, 199–201

Erotic overtures, in therapy, 118
as distortion, 105–109
as unhealthy well-being operation, 70

Etiology
of patient's pain, 48–51
preconceptions about, 10–12
of relationship distortions, 63, 92, 103–105

Evaluation, need for rapid, 8, 143–144

Existential group psychotherapy, 166–179

Expectations, in relationships, 153–157. *See also* Preconceptions

Exploratory group
  psychotherapy, 165–166
Extra-pyramidal syndromes
  (EPS), and antipsychotic
  medications, 186–187

Families, 2–3
  advice to, 151
  finding out about patient's,
    11–12, 76
  support for therapy by,
    128–130, 185, 190
Finding out, 6–8
  causes of pain, 48–53
  and interpretation, 67–69,
    81–87
  methods of, 12–19,
    142–144, 152–153
  other sources of patient
    data, 45–48, 51
Formulations. *See* Hypotheses
Future, patient's, 100, 138–140

Genomes, influence on
  personality, 33, 79
Group psychotherapy,
  problem-oriented,
    165–179
Guilt, 23, 92–94

Hedonism, discussion in
  existential groups, 176
History, patient's
  assumptions based on, 6–7,
    10–11
  finding out, 141–145,
    152–153
  misverifications in, 84–85
  other people's perspectives
    on, 11–12, 47, 148

and perception, 46–48,
  146–150
unconscious selection of,
  10–11, 124–125
Humor, use in therapy,
  114, 134–138,
  155–156
Hypotheses
  about patient behaviors,
    81–87
  in problem-oriented
    psychotherapy, 35–36

Identification, as well-being
  operation, 60–61
Information, therapist giving,
  75, 121
  through questions, 12, 14
Inspirational group
  psychotherapy, 166, 190
Interpersonal acts. *See*
  Relationships
Interpretations, therapist's,
  19, 51, 83
  example of, 44–45
Interviews
  deteriorating
    communication in,
      125–130
  organization of, 7–8,
    17–19, 141–146
Introductory words, for
  questions, 14–15
Involved sharing
  and observation, 158–159
  of psychotherapist and
    patient, 1–6, 81–82
Irrelevancies, 67, 118–119
  to block anxiety, 34,
    40–42

Legal actions, and medications, 187–188, 201
Lithium treatment, for manic disorders, 183, 188

Manic disorders, 87, 185
lithium for, 183, 188
medications for, 182, 195, 197, 202
Marxism, 158–161, 170–171
Meaning
of dreams, 132
of psychological terms, 8–10
Medications
antipsychotic, 85, 87
glossary of, 194–205
for treating emotional disorders, 181–193
Mental health profession. *See* Psychotherapy
Mind, concept of, 24–29, 89

Needs, in relationships, 153–157
Neuroses
causes of, 99, 101
medications for, 183–184, 188–189, 198
Noises, as nonverbal communication, 10–11, 124
Nonverbal communication, 14, 121–125
judging significance by, 33–34
selecting data through, 10–11, 124–125

Observable behaviors, 78
and energy flows, 90–91
in problem-oriented psychotherapy, 112, 157–163
Obsessions and compulsions
medications for, 198–199
as unhealthy energy flows, 92–96
as unhealthy well-being operations, 62, 65–67
Organization, of interviews, 7–8, 17–19, 141–146

Pain. *See also* Emotions
blocking therapy, 16, 19
and communication, 39–54
reduced through well-being operations, 56, 58, 62
from therapy, 8, 49, 98–99
Paranoia, as distortion in relationship, 102–103
Parenting, 91, 92. *See also* Families
Parkinsonism, and medications, 187, 195–198
Passivity, and patient's self-image, 8–9
Perception, 21–37, 85
pain as obstacle to, 45–48
Perceptive inattention, as well-being operation, 57–59
Personality, 8–10, 77–79, 91
formation of, 32–33, 60–61
of therapists, 114–118
Personality disorders, 183–184, 188–189

causes of, 99, 101, 103
Postponing discussions, 34,
    49, 52–53
    when anxiety gets too high,
    16, 41–42, 96
Praising therapists, as
    unhealthy well-being
    operation, 71
Preconceptions
    observer's, 159–160
    patient's, 6–8, 130
    therapist's, 10–12
Problem-oriented
    psychotherapy, 103–104
    goals of, 32–37
    with groups, 165–179
    observation in, 112,
    157–163
    principles of, 7–12, 69, 75
    procedures of, 12–19, 24,
    29–32, 81–87
Psychosis, 96, 99
    and antipsychotic
    medications, 182–189,
    194–205
    psychotherapy for, 85–87
Psychotherapists
    behaviors that affect
    patients, 111–118
    unhealthy well-being
    operations directed at, 9,
    67–71
Psychotherapy
    concept of the mind in,
    26–29
    with groups, 165–179
    medications in, 181–205
    preconceptions about, 6–7,
    8

previous experiences in,
    144, 153
tasks of, 37, 46, 132

Questions, in problem-
    oriented psychotherapy,
    8, 12–19, 150
    in initial interviews,
    142–144

Regression, as unhealthy
    well-being operation,
    64
Relationships, 15, 27–28, 37,
    53–54
    effect of therapy on,
    128–130
    energy flows in, 90–100
    eroticizing, 105–109
    in group therapy, 165–179
    patterns in, 32–36, 81–84,
    103–105
    with therapist, 9, 69,
    101–103
    threefold nature of,
    153–157, 161–162
    well-being operations in,
    55–57, 76–77
Religion, in existential
    groups, 168–172
Repetitiveness, 19, 144. *See
    also* Obsessions and
    compulsions

Safety, through indirect
    questions, 15–16
Schizophrenia, 87
    medications for, 182–186,
    194–205

Science
    as basis of psychotherapy,
        13–14, 24–29, 99–100,
        160–161
    and energy flows, 90–91
    lack in dream work,
        130–133
    vs. religion, 168–170, 172
Sedatives. *See* Sleeplessness
Self-image
    patient's, 146–150
    society's, 163–164
Sex
    dysfunction in, 42–45
    energy flows in, 91
    in group discussion,
        173–174
Sharing. *See also* Involved
        sharing
    with psychotherapists *vs.*
        laypeople, 2–6
Silence, significance of, 34–35
Sleeplessness, 92
    medications for, 190–193,
        194–205
Smith, Adam, 158–160
Society, problem-oriented
        psychotherapy on,
        157–164
Statements, 12, 18. *See also*
        Information, therapist
        giving
Sublimation, as well-being
        operation, 59–60
Suicide, 8, 143, 166–170
Summaries, 16. *See also*
        Interpretations
    after initial interviews,
        143–145

Symptoms
    as source of patient data,
        48
    as unhealthy well-being
        operations, 62

Tardive dyskinesia (TD),
        and antipsychotic
        medications, 187
Tendencies, cognitive, 48
Termination
    fears of, 104
    steps toward, 129–130
Third-party technique,
        75–77
Tourette's syndrome,
        medications for, 198
Training, for therapists, 34,
        70, 125
Transference, and problem-
        oriented psychotherapy,
        69, 70, 103–104

Understanding
    pain as obstacle to, 45–48
    psychotherapists
        ascertaining, 8–9

Verification, of hypotheses,
        81–87
Voice tones, 11, 13–14,
        124

Well-being operations, 55–79
Withdrawal, from
        relationships, 62–63,
        81–84
Words, use of psychological,
        8–10, 13–14